NAKED FITNESS

NAKED FITNESS

The Proven 28 Day
Weight Loss Program
for a Slimmer, Fitter,
Pain Free Body

Andrea Metcalf

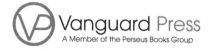

Vanguard Press
A Member of the Perseus Books Group

Copyright © 2010 by Andrea Metcalf

Published by Vanguard Press
A Member of the Perseus Books Group

Design and production by Eclipse Publishing Services
Set in 11.5-point Adobe Garamond

Cataloging-in-Publication data for this book is available
from the Library of Congress.

ISBN: 978-1-59315-618-3
Library of Congress Control Number: 2010936255

Vanguard Press books are available at special discounts for bulk purchases in the U.S. by corporations, institutions, and other organizations. For more information, please contact the Special Markets Department at the Perseus Books Group, 2300 Chestnut Street, Suite 200, Philadelphia, PA 19103, or call (800) 810-4145, ext. 5000, or e-mail special.markets@perseusbooks.com.

10 9 8 7 6 5 4 3 2 1

To my dad, who inspired me to be the best,
and to all my clients and everyone who has sought my advice
because they, too, wanted to be the best.

ACKNOWLEDGMENTS

I wish to thank my uniquely individual children: Bruce, Maddie, and Charlie, as well as Bruce, who was my partner for 20+ years. The four of them allowed me time to dedicate my life to my passion of health and fitness. I'm also very grateful to my mom and sisters for their constant love.

Thanks also to Lynnette K., Sue W., Mrs. B., Gina, Carolyn, Jamie B., Maggie G., and Rich M., who supported me and listened to my many hours of Naked chatter. To Brenda, Baltazar, Larry "Little Joe," PR Lou, mbc Fitness, Carmine, Richard Bux, Dixie Baker, Branko, Walter, Ann V., Jennifer W., Neil Sant, Roger, and Mike Burton for their constant support and feedback and to everyone at Vanguard Press for their support. I wrote *Naked Fitness* for all of you and for all the future friends I hope to inspire. To everyone: Feel good in your own skin and look good naked.

CONTENTS

NAKED FITNESS

The
Bare
Essence

1

WHAT IS NAKED FITNESS?

Naked Fitness."

I know you're thinking, "What is that? Does it mean I have to work out in the nude? Prance around in my birthday suit?"

The very idea of revealing your goods can be utterly terrifying. The primary reason is one that many of us likely have in common: the need to lose some weight. No one wants to strut around in the nude with a stomach that's far from flat or thighs that are nothing close to trim.

Let me reassure you: Naked Fitness isn't about working out in the nude or exercising in skimpy spandex for all the world to see. No, none of that.

Naked Fitness is about stripping away all the obstacles, barriers, and excuses in your life that keep you from getting your wonderful body into the best shape possible. It's about seeing how beautiful your real body is—an ever-evolving work of art—and feeling good about your body just as it is. The truth is that with a great body comes great confidence—with clothes or without them.

Naked Fitness is also about following a special, tailored-for-you nutrition and workout plan—one that will help you achieve a body worthy of complete exposure. And it's a plan you'll want to stay on and make a part of your lifestyle.

Yes, I'm sure you've taken the I-will-get-in-shape oath before. But maybe you didn't follow through. Maybe you tried to crash-diet your way down and got burned out in the process. Maybe you didn't give it your best shot. Or maybe you just didn't have a realistic game plan to ensure your success.

But now things are going to be different. You're going to be ready because you will have the right plan, and you are going to go about it in the right way, with a 28-day strategy for getting great results and looking your bare best.

I know Naked Fitness gets results, and I want to pass those on to you. In 2010, I selected 30 people from a group of 200 applicants to participate in my 28-day Naked Fitness program in my hometown of Chicago. Participants had to be at least 30 pounds overweight, have their doctor's consent, and be willing to attend a group support meeting every Saturday for a month. I instructed them to follow my simple Naked Fitness Nutrition Plan, perform a short daily strength and stretching program, and get in two hours of walking a day.

The results were phenomenal. The top "losers" in the program lost 20, 26, and 28 pounds, respectively, in just under a month. On average, weight loss was a whopping 18 pounds in a month! And collectively, the group that completed the challenge lost 491 pounds in four weeks. But those aren't the only numbers that changed. Participants saw healthy drops in blood pressure, cholesterol, triglycerides, heart rates, and fat to lean muscle ratios. Many people were relieved of their aches and pains and felt emotionally stronger.

No matter how much weight you have to lose—10 pounds, 15 pounds, 20 pounds, 50 or more pounds—this program is for everyone, not just those who are drastically overweight. And even if you just need to tone up, you can do that too—in as little as 15 minutes a day. I'll also introduce you to some new movement techniques that will help you approach getting in shape as a positive experience that will help guarantee success. You'll feel better than ever too, because unlike many exercise programs, Naked Fitness focuses on the alleviation of pain. You'll feel more flexible, more agile, and infinitely more youthful!

There is staying power in Naked Fitness, too. Most people who follow my Naked Fitness program find that they can easily stay on it and keep going, well beyond the initial 28-day period.

For example, Mike weighed more than 400 pounds prior to starting Naked Fitness. I had to use two scales to monitor his progress because a common bathroom scale only goes up to 350 pounds and he was much larger than that. Each week, I had him step on the scales three times, and I'd average the number in order to accurately record his results. And what results they were: Mike lost a personal record of 100 pounds in just 90 days, something he had never done before. He continues to lose more weight living the Naked Fitness lifestyle still. In Mike's own words, "Losing the weight brought back the swagger in my step."

Gina shed 135 pounds, but as important, she went off all her medication for diabetes and high blood pressure. At her recent physical, Gina's doctor even pronounced her diabetes "cured" as a result of the dietary and lifestyle changes she had made.

Lynn was able to reduce her total cholesterol from 282 to 230 and her LDL cholesterol (the artery-clogging kind) from 194 to 131—in only three months. Lynn's doctor predicts she will soon be able to stop taking all of her cholesterol-lowering medications.

Alan, a participant in the 28 days program, lost 26 pounds—almost 10 percent of his total body weight. He continued following the Naked Fitness program on his own, and four weeks later, he had lost another 14 pounds.

These are just a few of the amazing examples of what Naked Fitness can do. This program is so easy, doable, and maintainable that you will, perhaps for the first time ever, succeed and reach your health and fitness goals.

Once you get started on Naked Fitness, don't be surprised if, before you know it, you really do want to take it all off!

Here's a closer look at my Naked Fitness philosophy and what to expect.

Overcome Obstacles and Look Your Bare Best

One of the chief reasons we have so much trouble getting in shape and staying in shape is that life doesn't always follow that yellow-brick road Dorothy danced down. Sometimes it's more like an expressway after winter, full of potholes and bumps. There's always a pothole where you'd least expect it. And sometimes without warning, you suffer a blowout.

I experience these bumps and blowouts often, usually in the middle of the afternoon. A big bump for me is my craving for gummy candies, especially when I think I need a boost or a treat to make myself feel better. I'll rationalize that it's better to have a few pieces than to eat an ice cream sundae (which is true). But why am I really craving them in the first place? Even though I'm in the fitness business, I'm human. I have imperfections. I crave sugar when I'm stressed out, tired, bored, or lonely. It's just one of those obstacles that I have to strip away.

Naked Fitness is about doing just that: stripping away stuff like unhealthy, toxic habits, negative thinking, cravings, lack of time to exercise, emotional overeating, people who sabotage you, poor self-esteem and body image, and one of the biggest obstacles of all: stress. With these factors managed or out of your life completely, you are guaranteed to lose weight and keep it off. Plus, you'll boost your "naked confidence," a love-your-body attitude that will improve your life as a whole.

Align Yourself

Many people think being fit is a function of how much toned muscle and how little body fat they have. And that's true, but it's not the whole story. What they often don't realize is that proper postural alignment is the key to looking younger and thinner, as well as to improving your health and well-being. For best results from an exercise program, you need balanced muscles that are the correct length and strength to equalize the forces around your joints. Muscle imbalances occur because of repeated movement. Some muscles get shorter and stronger in relationship to others that become longer and weaker. The shorter, stronger muscles get too stiff from overworking and pull the forces around your joints off-center, while other areas of your body compensate and become too flexible. The ideal situation is one in which your body segments are balanced in the position of optimal alignment and maximum support, with full mobility available.

The key difference between my program and others is that we work on and correct postural alignment. I'll show you how to self-evaluate your alignment and give you daily personalized strength and stabilizing exercises to bring your entire body back into alignment. This is essential. Unless you correct your postural alignment, the effectiveness of your training is diminished and you may become more prone to injury. By doing your alignment work, you set the stage for better and faster aesthetic results in the weeks to come.

Walk It Off

Walking is an easy, do-anywhere form of exercise. You can walk your dog. You can walk to work (well, not really if it's more than a few miles away from home). You can walk over to the printer. You can walk on a treadmill. Walking is the American Heart Association's recommended way to start an exercise program.

In Naked Fitness, I'll ask you to walk two hours each day. I know, this seems impossible, but take heart; you don't have to do it all at once. You can break your walking up into smaller, doable time chunks every day. The key is to get in two hours of walking a day—and trust me, you can lose as much weight, and as fast, as the participants in my Naked Fitness Chicago experiment did.

Although walking is an ability we take for granted, I'll teach you to walk in such a way that you burn calories more efficiently. Most people walk improperly; this distorts posture, can throw your bones and spine out of alignment, and can affect your muscles adversely. To get the most from walking, you'll follow my super-fun, stylized walking techniques called Walk-ilates™, such as heel walking, side walking, crossover walking, waist-whittler walking, and heel-to-toe rock. You'll learn a whole new way to walk. Mastering these techniques is well worth the effort, because the better your alignment, the more calories you burn.

There's more: Walking has also been shown to raise the metabolic rate for one to four hours after an exercise session, so you'll continue to expend energy and burn calories. And in another study, people who engaged in walking versus jogging stuck to their programs longer and lost more weight as a result.

There are many positive results to be gained from walking besides weight loss. At the top of the list are improved cardiovascular health, strengthened bones, stress reduction, and improved attitude and mental health.

The Naked Fitness Nutrition Plan

In addition to moving, good eating habits result in a body you can be proud of. On Naked Fitness, you'll eat according to my "naked nutrition" guidelines. This means eating more clean, vital, and energy-producing foods and fewer foods dressed in fat-laden sauces or laced with preservatives, added sugar, and other food junk.

Think of your body as a luxury car. You simply can't put junk in a car like that. It's not going to run smoothly. Starches, sugars, and processed foods clog up the body's engine, causing it to perform poorly. Naked nutrition, on the other hand, can rev up your metabolic engine and boost muscle, which helps burn body fat, plus result in fantastic energy levels and other benefits. Keep in mind that eating lots of junk can pack on pounds, which won't do your figure any favors in its naked state.

For weight loss, my naked nutrition guidelines follow a standard, tried-and-true equation: eat more + do less = weigh more; eat less + do more = weigh less. It doesn't matter who you are; this equation applies to everyone.

My friend Sue used to disagree with me on this. Even though she exercised, Sue would spend several days mindlessly eating bread and dessert, and had wine most nights of the week, and she wondered why she gained 10 pounds so quickly. I explained repeatedly to her that when we put junk in the fuel tank, junk in the trunk (and elsewhere) is the result. Living mindlessly leads to weight gain and poor health.

Eventually, Sue set her mind to living more healthfully. She paid attention to what she ate. She began eating more fruits and vegetables and cut down on the amount of high-fat foods in her diet. She ate smaller portions and, most important, stopped eating when she felt satisfied. She told me, "I didn't feel like I had to stuff myself to the point where I could barely breathe." Over the next few months, her clothes got looser, and she eventually lost 13 pounds. Sue's naked confidence skyrocketed, and she liked her body better, even when stark naked.

I learned long ago to base my dietary preferences on this one question: How will I feel if I eat this food? After much experimentation, I have found that I feel best when my diet consists of plenty of water, fruit, vegetables, yogurt, nuts, lean meat, and fish. At 40+ years of age, I have decided to put less sugar, preservatives, flour, gluten, alcohol, and unhealthy fats in my body. The difference in how I look and feel is so profound that I want everyone to eat this way—the naked nutrition way.

The Naked Fitness Nutrition Plan isn't really a diet, because it doesn't deprive you or leave you famished. When you deprive yourself, what's actually showing up on the scale is a loss of muscle weight. Why is that such a big deal? Muscle tissue is one of the largest contributing factors in determining the speed of your metabolism. So when your body is forced to burn its own muscle for energy, it sets off a chain reaction of detrimental consequences such as fat storage.

The Naked Fitness Nutrition Plan also shows you how to incorporate many of the foods you and your family usually eat. After about two weeks of following my guidelines, naked nutrition will become so second nature to you that you'll be able to easily select your own foods, prepare them, and eat your way to a beautifully naked body!

Group Support

Study after study shows that anyone who has a support group—family or friends, an organized gathering, or even someone they hire—cheering them on is more successful with long-term weight loss than people who try to go it alone. In fact, if you have support, you are 70 percent more likely to make positive changes, but with no support, your odds drop to only 9 percent for losing weight and keeping it off. Research shows that one person in ten is successful in achieving weight loss goals when going it alone. A support group can help you keep weight off over the long term and keep you connected and motivated.

You'll want to locate a support group where everyone has a chance to participate, the mood is upbeat, and you feel comfortable. This can be an online support group, too, which can be invaluable. Join the www.nakedfitness.com online support team, where you will receive additional recipes, exercises, and motivational messages and be able to share your stories. Or you can team up with friends and do Naked Fitness together and then form your own support group. What will help you is hearing other people's stories and sharing recipes and menus and advice on how to manage your diet and your weight.

Another recommendation is to do your exercises and walking with a partner. Exercise brings any relationship to a different intensity due to the hormonal changes that happen while you're working out with another person. Both of you will see results in just a few weeks of training, plus strengthen your friendship bond.

With support, you'll have a whole group of people cheering you on. You don't have to do this alone.

Believe You Can Lose It

All our past experiences mold our current thinking and actions. Many people, for example, think they can't lose weight, either because of their "slow" metabolisms, their mothers' large thighs, or because they've had trouble sticking with diets or exercise routines in the past. This kind of thinking is what I call "ANTs," shorthand for "another negative thought." ANTs have to be stomped out—and I'll give you the tools to do it.

Why is it so crucial to curb negative thoughts? They can have a negative effect on other areas of your life and snowball into "I'm not doing well at work," "I won't go to that party," "I'm not desirable," and basically wear down your self-esteem. I will help you stop the self-sabotage.

Not long ago, I worked with Leah, 38-year-old working (and traveling) mother of two children, both under the age of 6. She confessed that she had always lacked discipline and was a self-proclaimed "junk-food junkie." As a result, her weight ballooned and she kept having to buy larger and larger sizes. Leah's biggest problem, though, wasn't lack of exercise and poor eating. It was her mind. She kept telling herself this ANT: "My weight will never change; it is what my body became after having children."

So we had to work on stripping away those thoughts, replacing them with positive mantras, and designing a program that fit Leah's on-the-go lifestyle and included hotel workouts. Once all the pieces fell into place, Leah began shedding pounds at the rate of a pound a week. Before long, she had lost a healthy ten pounds and tossed out all her fat clothes. She has not gained back one ounce.

As Leah found, once you believe success is possible, you'll feel less intimidated by any challenges and temptations that come your way. Losing weight and getting fitter is like planting a little seed in the ground. You provide a warm, lighted environment and water it daily. Nothing much happens for about 10 days. Then, suddenly, a wonderful, healthy green plant begins to emerge. In a few months, you might have a flower or a fruit. Change is like that—a growing experience—and it takes time. You will start feeling wonderful, and you will want to show off those gains you achieved with Naked Fitness. Being in great physical condition allows you to be much more confident about yourself, and I believe that if you feel good about your physique, you will have more energy, better relationships, and more self-confidence in everything you do.

Put Yourself First

Before you even get started, I want you to decide you are worth the effort. Make your health and fitness your number one priority. What does that mean? It means that before every decision you make, ask yourself, "What is the healthiest choice I can make?" It also means that you have permission to be selfish, because you are important, worthy, satisfied, and wonderful.

These days, life is complex. Most of us—me included—juggle the numerous hats modern-day society requires us to wear. Married or single, we have multiple roles as parent, spouse, maid, cook, nurse, tutor, and chauffeur, coupled with full-time employment demands. The demands of "role-overload" can leave us feeling overwhelmed, stressed out, and anxious if we're not careful. And consistently having too much to do in too little time can anger and depress us, rendering us of little use to anyone, especially to ourselves. We have to make an effort to shield ourselves from these potentially debilitating emotions. My solution is to put myself first, strive for more balance, and be more assertive about seeking support and asking for help. When you put yourself first, you take care of yourself, both mentally and physically. This makes you a better parent, spouse, employee, and so forth.

I once surveyed a group of men and women, and I asked them, "Do you do something for yourself every day?" About 56 percent of the women and 68 percent of the men said they did something to take care of themselves every day. One lady's comment was interesting: "Now that I am 50, it's time to take care of me. So yes, I do something just for me every day."

I wondered why she waited so long! You should be doing something for yourself every day from birth forward. You are the priority.

So take a closer look at yourself and ask, "Do you deserve to be healthy?" "Do you want to be healthy?" and lastly, "Do you believe that your body is your best asset?" I have asked these questions of myself, and my answer is a resounding YES! I want balance in my life and want to feel good about myself. These emotions drive my health regimen and help me feel fulfilled in my own naked body.

Please let this be the time you put yourself first. It's time to make yourself a priority and get your game into gear. Get active, toss out your excuses, and get an added edge with Naked Fitness.

Getting Naked

If you're tired of being unhappy with your weight and not doing anything about it, you have come to the right place. The fact that you've picked up this book tells me that you're aware of your current situation, that you no longer want to live the way you've been living, and you know something must change. My hope is that you'll keep this book handy as a guide and motivator. There are some wonderful tools in the appendices to help you. It has been my goal to make the information easy to understand, easy to find, and easy to use.

Using this practical, results-oriented plan, you'll learn how to get your body in shape—and feel great about yourself at the same time. Just think: No more angst in front of the fitting room mirror as you stare at yourself and shake your head over how flabby you look. No more dreaded days of reckoning in which you must wriggle into a bathing suit. No more feeling so self-conscious that you have to camouflage your hips and thighs with baggy dresses and pants. No more. Not ever again.

I'll show you how to get in control of your body and achieve your goals so you can be the person you want to be. Naked Fitness can help you look and feel like the sexy, attractive person you are and give you an added advantage so you can achieve your weight-loss goals like never be-fore. Exercise and nutrition will become fun because you'll start to see how your body is changing for the better. You'll suddenly start having good thoughts about your body and more confidence in yourself. For the first time in years, you won't mind wearing a bathing suit or other body-baring outfits. The sensation of showing off your body will be amazing. No longer do you have to let your shape—or your appraisal of it—run your life.

Naked Fitness will help you be happy about and proud of what you have, naked or otherwise. Ready to change? Read on.

2

FACING THE MIRROR

Do you like what you see in the mirror? Do you have that constant negative message: "I'm too much of this. . . too little of that. . . ?" Do you like your shape this year, but last year you could barely look at it? How do you feel about your body, honestly?

I once interviewed 60 people (28 men and 32 women) to see whether they like their bodies naked, among other questions. For the most part, the group was comprised of school administrators from Colorado, aged approximately 25 to 60, of all different body sizes and shapes.

There were many laughs, giggles, red faces, and shoulder shrugs, depending on whether they were asked individually or as part of a group. (The group interviews drew the most giggles.) Of the men, 16, or 57 percent, said they liked their bodies naked. Of the women, only 14, or 43 percent, said they liked their bodies naked. So generally, the guys seemed to like their naked bodies better than the women did. One man told me, "I see all my muscles in the mirror. Although some aren't as developed as they used to be, I focus only on the ones that are, and I am happy with what I see."

Women, on the other hand, seem to see only what they don't like, as in "Isn't that gross? This bounces. This sags." Honestly, I can relate: Like when I wear jeans and my softness spills over the waistline into that so-called "muffin-top" (whoever coined that term, down with them!).

Can a low opinion of your body affect how you perceive yourself in other areas of your life? Can it affect your success at getting in shape and regaining your health? Definitely. If you don't like your body, you are apt not to like yourself—and not to take good care of your health.

You and your body are one. When you're nice to it, nourishing it with healthy foods and energizing it with exercise, your body feels appreciated, works well, and helps you reach your health and weight-loss goals. But when you mistreat your body, punishing it by calling it "fat," or medicating sadness with junk food pig-outs, you give it no reason to perform the way you want it to, which only reinforces your negative thoughts and bad treatment.

However, don't despair. You can overcome the obstacles to loving your body, improve your body image, and get in great shape permanently.

Bare All!

How can you start to feel good about the way you look? By looking in the mirror! Take off your clothes and stand in front of a full-length mirror in bright light! Really see what's in the reflection.

I'll admit that making friends with your full-length looking glass isn't easy (especially under fluorescent lights in a swimsuit-store dressing room). At age 55, Madelyn, one of my clients, told me the only time she looks in the mirror is when she brushes her teeth, puts on makeup, or does her hair. If she catches a glimpse of herself walking out of the shower, she quickly turns away, not wanting to see the body that has changed so much over the years.

But the more you look, the less you'll stress. So face that fear—literally. Avoiding looking at your nude body in the mirror just leads to more emotional anxiety. Think of it as like falling off a bike: If you have a bad experience and refuse to try again, your mind will blow it up into something much scarier than it really was. To get the wheels turning, you need to desensitize yourself to strip down anxiety.

If you're particularly squeamish, it's okay to wear just your undies. Our goal isn't to become the next nudist-camp member; it's just to get you comfortable with your bare body.

So take a look and be honest about your body. Everyone essentially has the same one. We are made up of arms, legs, a torso, a head, about 350 bones, and 600 dying-to-be-toned muscles. So why do we all look so different? The answer is not solely genetics. It's all the experiences we have encountered that change and shape our physique. For example, carrying a 22-pound backpack of books in sixth grade. Sitting at the computer for two hours a day answering emails. Running five miles a day for a couple of decades. Sleeping four hours a night. Standing in the airport security line for 45 minutes several times a month. The sports we played. Wearing shoes with poor support year after year. All of that and more. Every activity that we have engaged in voluntarily or not has left a mark on our movement patterns, body alignment, and possibly even our bone structure.

Take a good, realistic look at every inch of your body. It's you! I bet you'll find it's not as bad as you think. The most incredible news is that you have the power to change just about any feature you care to. And you also have the power to love just about any part of your body. By loving yourself and taking care of your body and mind, you'll be taking better care of your health.

Seven Secrets to Loving Your Body, Naked or Otherwise

In this age where taut, toned limbs seem to command more respect than an advanced degree, it's no small wonder that it has become extremely hard for people to feel good about their bodies. Learning to love your body is not impossible. All you need are the right tools. Here are some steps to help you.

1. DETERMINE A REALISTIC WEIGHT FOR YOU

Instead of striving for physical perfection, developing a positive body image demands turning your focus—and your time—to health. This requires taking into account your genetic predispositions and age and the amount of time you have to devote to your realistic weight. Decide on a healthy weight that you can achieve—not an impossible one guaranteed to bring on disappointment. It could be a mental snapshot from the past, such as when you were a size 10 before having kids, or a weight at which you were comfortable, such as your weight when you were in college or when you got married.

There is really no such thing as the perfect weight because we are all different. There are, however, healthy weight ranges, and you can determine these through a very simple calculation: Take 100 pounds for the first five feet of your height and add five pounds for each extra inch to get the midpoint of what should be your ideal body weight range.

If you fall within 10 percent on either side (lower or higher) of that midpoint, you are within your ideal weight range. The lower end of the ranges are for small-boned individuals; the upper end, for larger-boned people. Look through the chart on page 19. It shows ideal weight ranges (with the midpoints in bold).

Your physician can also help you set healthy and realistic weight-loss goals.

2. IDENTIFY AREAS FOR CHANGE

If you're not completely satisfied with your body, what would you change? Pick any and all parts or part that you would like to be different. Pick them now! How would you like these areas to be different? Smaller arms, longer-looking legs, fuller bottom, or is it that you just want to move freely without pain or the reminder of aging. How small or big are the changes? The deeper the ditch, the more you must dig. But remember, you can dig deeper and wider, and there are no limits to how much earth you can move, only how much dirt you can move in one day. You can have the body you desire. Once you've identified areas you'd like to be different, better, smaller, or bigger, list them in a journal. Writing it down creates awareness and accountability. Your attitude will start to change because you gave those problem parts more care than you usually would. You'll relax more and be less judgmental about your perceived flaws.

3. FIND SOMETHING TO LOVE

While looking at your reflection, find parts of your body you like. What I try to help people do is just look, not make any judgments; in effect, just say, "That is me." Then I encourage them to focus on only the things they like—and why.

For example, I'll have them name a positive function for each body part or muscle: "My arms are strong enough to carry my child." "My legs allow me to run, and I feel good when I do that."

This exercise will remind you how crucial your body's physical performance is to your existence and is a good one to try if you just can't seem to see beyond how big your thighs look in shorts. Or if your hateful gaze is always directed toward your midsection, intercept the insults by saying something positive and true aloud, such as "This is the stomach that stretched to support my babies while they grew healthy and strong inside me."

Still having trouble finding something to love? If it isn't a body part, then maybe it's the way you handle others, care for others, lead or direct others, or some other amazing talent you have. Love yourself for it. Accept what makes you unique. When you believe in yourself, you gain a sense of control that helps you succeed in life. Embracing yourself in this way will help you make changes that will last a lifetime.

4. AFFIRM YOURSELF DAILY

Start each day with the reminder that, yes, you are wonderful. Your body is uniquely and magnificently yours. List all the gorgeous or handsome things about your body on Post-it notes and stick one on your bathroom mirror each morning.

I am a big believer in affirmations, mantras, and positive sayings. Setting out to lose weight, get in shape, or improve your health requires a certain mindset. If you decide that health is the way you're going to live, then set it in motion by using positive affirmations. Some of my favorite sayings are listed on pages 22 and 23.

Do not underestimate the power of these seemingly simple tips. If you're reading any of these and thinking, "Yeah, yeah, positive thinking. I know this already," but you're not practicing these principles, then you really DO NOT know, and you don't understand how vitally important it really is.

5. VISUALIZE YOUR SUCCESS

Form the image of your healthy body in your mind. In your mind's eye, see yourself at your healthy, realistic weight, fitting into a dress two sizes smaller than you wear now or moving with ease. Then, in a simple journal or on the sheet in Appendix C called Steps to My Healthy Body, describe your healthy body and write down actions you can take to actualize it. These might include losing 15 pounds, exercising more, learning to rock climb, eating more vegetables, making Naked Fitness your lifestyle, or all of the above.

When visualizing, you form vivid pictures in your conscious mind. Those pictures of your goals or objectives are kept alive until they sink into your subconscious mind. When they reach the subconscious mind, untapped energies are released to help visualized pictures become reality.

A lot of people think of visualizations as something practiced only by high-performance athletes, but they can do wonders for the everyday exerciser as well. Because visualizations require a certain degree of relaxation, the naturally mellow periods after you've just woken up or before you go to bed are perfect times to start. Give yourself the power to see that shapely, gracefully moving body. Close your eyes and see yourself being there now, having those changes completed right now.

While Mike was in the process of losing 100 pounds in 90 days, he used visualization to help him. At week six, he had shed about 50 pounds, and his clothes were falling off him. His waistline was in the 50-inch range. I commented, "Just wait until you are a 34-inch waistline!"

At first, he didn't believe he could do it. I encouraged him to keep visualizing, if not a 34-inch waist, a healthy body. I told him that when he achieved a healthy weight and body, a side effect would be a 34-inch waist.

Mike amped up his visualizations. A few weeks later, sure enough, he was wearing 34 x 30 jeans. What you believe, you will achieve.

6. BE KIND TO YOURSELF

Place copies of one of your childhood photos in your desk drawer, on your fridge door, or by your computer. When you see the image, remind yourself that the little person is still you. Then vow to be nicer to her. Stop telling her she doesn't deserve to be happy until she loses 20 pounds. You'd never treat your own kids that way, so you need to be more nurturing toward your most vulnerable self in the present day.

When you constantly put down your body with a certain phrase (for example, "I'm a blob"), that belief becomes imprinted in your brain, so you actually begin to move like you're a blob. Build a more positive body-image identity: Immediately replace hurtful insults with a phrase that captures a trait you love about yourself that's not body-related; for example, "I am confident," or "I am a loving friend." You may not believe your new phrase immediately, but over time you can convince yourself to feel more positive.

7. MAKE A CONSCIOUS COMMITMENT TO CHANGE

Like all health-promoting activities, creating a body that looks and feels good naked requires lifestyle changes. It doesn't begin simply with an exercise prescription, a calculated recommended body weight, or a session with a personal trainer. To think of redesigning the body only in physical terms would be superficial and temporary. Redesigning your body means rethinking every aspect of the body mentally, emotionally, spiritually, physiologically, and physically. It begins with how you feel about your body and is followed by knowing and appreciating how your body is made, how it works, and what you must do to enable it to function most efficiently and effectively.

Rethink your body with the goal of having the best body possible. Begin to love your unique and magnificent body so much that you want to present your best body to the world. Your best body is your "beautiful" body. It is achieved by attaining your best percent body fat, your best weight, your best blood pressure reading, and your best cholesterol reading. Your best body may look different from people you admire, but it is your best body.

34 POSITIVE SAYINGS

- Be healthy and be moved. — *Andrea Metcalf*
- Something's gotta give. — *Anonymous*
- If you believe you can or cannot, you are correct. — *Henry Ford*
- Cultivate the habit of laughter. — *Og Mandino*
- Your imagination is your preview of life's coming attractions. — *Albert Einstein*
- You can't fail if you don't give up. — *Anonymous*
- Wish well, be well. — *Turkish proverb*
- May all your dreams turn into goals. — *Catherine Pulsifer*
- Procrastination is the fear of success. — *Denis Waitley*
- If one dream should fall and break into a thousand pieces, never be afraid to pick one of those pieces up and begin again. — *Flavia Weedn*
- Go confidently in the direction of your dreams. Live the life you have imagined. — *Henry David Thoreau*
- When you feel like giving up, remember why you held on for so long in the first place. — *Anonymous*
- Risk more than others think is safe. Care more than others think is wise. Dream more than others think is practical. Expect more than others think is possible. — *Claude Bissell*
- Never let the odds keep you from doing what you know in your heart you were meant to do. — *H. Jackson Brown, Jr.*
- A diamond is merely a lump of coal that did well under pressure. — *Anonymous*
- You have to expect things of yourself before you can do them. — *Michael Jordan*
- I always felt that my greatest asset was not my physical ability; it was my mental ability. — *Bruce Jenner*
- The purpose of life is a life of purpose. — *Robert Byrne*
- Physical fitness is not only one of the most important keys to a healthy body; it is the basis of dynamic and creative intellectual activity. — *John F. Kennedy*

34 POSITIVE SAYINGS (continued)

- Work like you don't need money. Love like you've never been hurt, and dance like no one's watching. — *Aurora Greenway*

- It's never too late to be what you might have been. — *George Eliot*

- Those who do not find time for exercise will have to find time for illness. — *Earl of Derby*

- It is remarkable how one's wits are sharpened by physical exercise. — *Pliny the Younger*

- Movement is a medicine for creating change in a person's physical, emotional, and mental states. — *Carol Welch*

- If you have an hour, will you not improve that hour, instead of idling it away? — *Lord Chesterfield*

- Every day, do something that will inch you closer to a better tomorrow. — *Doug Firebaugh*

- Accept challenges, so that you may feel the exhilaration of victory. — *George S. Patton*

- Challenges are what make life interesting; overcoming them is what makes life meaningful. — *Joshua J. Marine*

- Failure is only the opportunity to begin again, this time more wisely. — *Anonymous*

- Great changes may not happen right away, but with effort even the difficult may become easy. — *Bill Blackman*

- When you get to the end of your rope, tie a knot and hang on. — *Franklin D. Roosevelt*

- Never, never, never give up. — *Winston Churchill*

- There is no pleasure in life equal to that of the conquest of a vicious habit. — *Anonymous*

- That first peak is the best place to pause and look back, to see if you took the easiest route, to learn the lessons from the first climb. And it is the best place to examine the terrain ahead, to change your plans and goals, to take a deep breath and begin climbing again. — *Michael Johnson*

How you feel about your naked body in the mirror affects what you do, where you want to be seen, what you wear, and ultimately how you feel. Get in the habit of looking in the mirror on a regular basis. Before long, you'll like what you see.

3

THE NAKED FITNESS
FIT TEST

If you really want to strut your stuff in your natural state, you've got to have a personalized program that takes into consideration your body, your alignment, and your health goals. The first step toward designing that program is to take my Naked Fitness Fit Test. It will lead to a program tailored to suit you and let you keep tabs on your progress over time.

Your program will be based primarily on how your body moves and is aligned. Everything we do involves alignment, whether catching the bus or working at a computer or hiking to the top of a mountain. Alignment is the key to effective movement and better health.

I learned this truth while in college at DePaul University. My kinesiology professor gave the class the assignment to go to a local park and watch people walk, jog, and run. As I sat there observing, I was struck by the number of walking wounded limping around or walking with choppy form. A few were moving with fluidity.

Why was this? As I eventually learned, it all had to do with alignment. Having poor alignment is one of the most common ways people develop a multitude of health problems. Simply having your hips in the wrong place, your chest concave, or your head positioned incorrectly can cause serious problems and a great deal of unnatural wear and tear on your body.

Additionally, bad alignment keeps your skeletal, respiratory, nervous, digestive, and circulatory systems from functioning properly. This dysfunction is damaging on many levels: It hurts your physical fitness, digestion, ability to deal with stress and illness, and even your cognition. In fact, bad alignment can inhibit all of your bodily systems, causing parts of your body to not receive enough oxygen, nutrients, or neural messages. Teaching people to improve their alignment has never been more urgent, due primarily to the sheer numbers who put themselves at risk for injury.

So let's analyze your alignment so that you can begin to function better and, of course, look fabulous naked. You may keep your clothes on for this assessment. Be honest as you answer the questions. You may want to work with a partner to help you be more accurate. There is a worksheet in Appendix D called Standing in the Mirror Naked that can help you with your answers.

Depending on your answers, you'll be matched to one of four very distinct alignment routines and a level at which to begin your Naked Fitness routine.

Part 1: Alignment Test

In each of the assessments, check the statement that best represents your observation.

SECTION A: STANDING POSITION

Stand in front of a mirror with your arms at your side and feet forward. Look at your body. Take a few moments to notice each part of your body and see which sentences hold true for you.

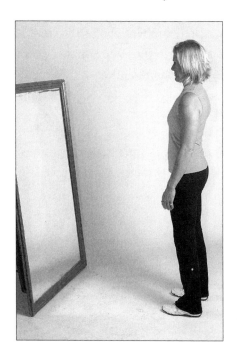

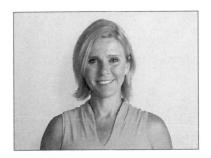

Your Head

Imagine a string dropping down from the top of your nose.
Answer the following:

The string lines up exactly in the center of the chest. ____ A

The string lines up slightly to the left or right. ____ B

One of my ears is higher than the other. ____ C

Your Shoulders

One of my shoulders is slightly higher than the other. ____ B

One of my shoulders is significantly higher than the other. ____ C

One or both of my shoulders round toward my chest. ____ C

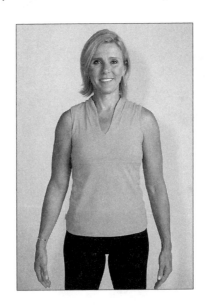

Your Palms

One or both of my hands face toward my hips. ____ B

One or both of my hands face forward. ____ A

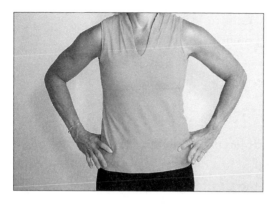

Your Hip Bones

Place your hands on your hips, with your index fingers on the bones in front.

My right side is higher than my left. ___ D

My left side is higher than my right. ___ D

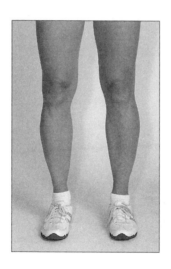

Your Knees

Looking at the top of my knee cap:

My knee caps are exactly even. ___ A

Both of my knee caps align directly over the centers of my feet. ___ A

One of my knee caps is higher than the other. ___ D

One of my knee caps or both lean to the outside. ___ D

One of my knee caps or both face somewhat to the inside. ___ D

Your Feet

Both of my feet point straight forward. ____ A

One of my feet or both point slightly to the outside. ____ D

One of my feet or both point slightly inward. ____ D

SECTION B: LYING DOWN

When your body lies parallel with gravity, the stress on your spinal structures is pulled in a different direction. No longer are the vertebrae being smashed together like lunch meat between two slices of bread. Instead, they are in a relaxed position. This section analyzes your alignment from a prone position.

Find a firm surface and/or carpeted area and lie down on your back, face up to the ceiling. Take a few moments to notice each part of your body and see which sentences hold true.

Your Head

My chin tilts up toward the ceiling. ____ B

My chin tilts toward my chest. ____ A

My chin points slightly to the side. ____ C

Your Shoulder Blades

My shoulder blades feel even on the ground. ____ A

There is more weight on one shoulder blade than on the other. ____ C

Your Palms

One or both of my palms face up. ____ A

One or both of my palms face down. ____ B

Your Buttocks Area

I feel evenly balanced on the ground.__ A

I feel more weight on one side of my behind than the other. ____ D

The backs of my thighs touch the ground. ____ A

The backs of my thighs do not touch the ground. ____ D

Your Knees

My knee caps are even and in the center of my legs. _____ A

One of my knee caps is higher than the other. ___ D

One of my knee cap faces somewhat to the outside. ___ D

One of my knee caps faces somewhat to the inside. ___ C

Your Feet

Both of my feet point straight up. ___ A

One or both of my feet point slightly to the outside. ___ D

One or both of my feet point slightly inward. ___ C

SECTION C: STANDING SQUAT

Stabilized positions like those above are an easy way to spot muscle imbalances and alignment issues. Movement, however, enables you to determine with a better degree of certainty where you might be misaligned. Here, I'll ask you to look at yourself while squatting— a position similar to one you do every day on the porcelain goddess.

Start with your hands over your head and your arms extended toward the ceiling. In one fluid motion, begin sitting back towards

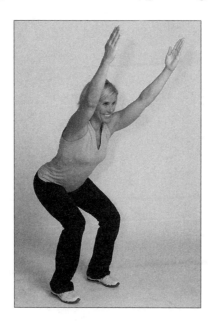

a chair in a squat position. Keep your arms extended and straight as much as possible and held as high as possible, each time you sit. Perform three squats and hold the final squat as you ask yourself the following questions.

Your Arms

My arms were inclined to bend at the elbow. ___ C

My arms stayed straight and could move above my ears. ___ A

My arms easily moved above my head but my elbows stayed bent. ___ C

My arms stayed straight but fell below my ears. ___ B

Your Head

My head stayed in place while I squatted. ___ A

My head lifted up while I squatted. ___ B

My head dropped to my chest while I squatted. ___ C

Your Hips

It was easy to sit back with my hips at 90 degrees. ___ A

My hips moved only to about 45 degrees. ___ C

My hips moved less than 45 degrees. ___ D

Your Knees

One or both of my knees leaned over my toes. ___ C

One or both of my knees moved out to the sides. ___ D

One or both of my knees stayed behind my toes. ___ A

One or both of my knees dropped in toward each other. ___ C

SECTION D: MY SHOE TEST

Walking is something I analyze with every client who walks through my door. But it's difficult to watch your own foot placement and stride. Instead, I want you to take a look at your most worn shoes. Find a pair of flats or gym shoes. Turn them over and looks at the soles. Identify signs of wear, in which most of the rubber has worn away. (If you don't have any shoes that show signs of wear, put yourself in the D category for this portion of the assessment.) Now, answer the following questions.

My shoes are worn mostly:
On the toes. ____ C
On the outside edges. ____ D
On the heel. ____ A
Not worn anywhere. ____ D

SECTION E: FLEXIBILITY

To perform this part of the test, you must be able to bend at the waist. If you can't, due to a previous injury, do not do this part. Instead, give yourself a D, which will help place you in the proper category as we move forward.

For safety and support, perform this exercise holding on to a chair or stool. Make sure your feet are parallel, about four to six inches apart,

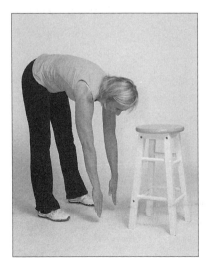
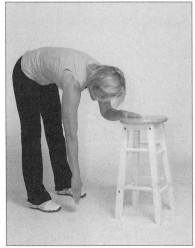

with your toes pointing forward. Keep your legs straight but do not lock your knees. Slowly bend at the waist and reach toward your toes. Use the stool for support if needed. Then return to the standing position. (If you cannot do this, please skip this part of the assessment and score yourself with a D.)

Which of the following statements is true for you?
I can easily touch my toes without bending my knees. ＿＿ A
I can easily touch my ankles without bending my knees. ＿＿ C
I can easily touch my shins without bending my knees. ＿＿ D
In general, it hurts to bend over, but I can touch my knees. ＿＿ D

SCORING FOR PART 1
To find your score, add up the number of A, B, C, and D answers.
- If your tally is mostly As, your alignment program will be the Cervical Spine (or Upper Back) Focus.
- If your tally is mostly Bs, your alignment program will be the Thoracic Spine (or Mid Back) Focus.
- If your tally is mostly Cs, your alignment program will be the Lumbar Spine (or Lower Back) Focus.
- If your tally is mostly Ds, your alignment program will be the Overall Body Focus.
- If you are unsure which routine to perform, perform routine D, Overall Body Focus.

Part 2: The Mile Test

In this part of my fitness assessment, we'll measure your aerobic fitness. Aerobic fitness is the ability to sustain physical activity for an extended period of time (as in running and biking) and is a measure of the health of our heart, lungs, and vascular system. When you hop on the treadmill or go out for a walk, you are performing aerobic exercise (also called cardiovascular exercise, or cardio). Most people participate in aerobic exercise in an effort to lose weight, burn body fat, and improve the health of their hearts.

You can measure your aerobic fitness with a simple walking test that can help not only track your progress against yourself but also in comparison to established norms for your age and gender. Here's how to begin.

- Find a measured, one-mile track at a school, park, or recreation center. If you want to measure a mile yourself, find a smooth, level surface. You can also do this test on a treadmill.

- Bring a stopwatch or a watch with a second hand, a pencil and paper, and comfortable walking shoes.

- Get your heart rate up to at least 110 beats per minute without straining. To check your heart rate, place two fingers in the groove in your neck that runs alongside your Adam's apple or on your wrist. Count the number of pulse beats in six seconds and add a zero. (This will give you your heartbeats per minute.) For example, if you count 12 pulse beats in six seconds, your heart rate is 120 beats per minute. You can also use a heart-rate monitor.

- Measure your pulse five minutes into your walk. Make sure your pulse remains above 110 beats per minute.

- Maintain a constant pace as you walk. Remember to keep your breathing smooth and regular.

- Record the time (in minutes and seconds) that it took to walk one mile. Most people take between 10 and 20 minutes to walk a mile.

- When you finish walking the mile, keep moving slowly and immediately take your pulse. Write this number down too.

- Continue to walk slowly for a few minutes to allow your heart rate and blood pressure to return to normal levels.

SCORING FOR PART 2

To score your test, find the chart for your sex, and then find your age range and your heart rate. If your exact pulse isn't shown, round it up or down to the nearest 10 beats.

Examples

- If you are a 47-year-old man who walked the one-mile course with a heart rate of 120 in 16 minutes, you would be at a moderate fitness level.

- If you are a 33-year-old woman who walked the course with a heart rate of 150 in 17 minutes, 30 seconds, you would also be at a moderate fitness level.

You've now established a baseline for your aerobic fitness based on two factors: the length of time it took you to complete the mile and your heart rate when you were done. You can repeat this test every six weeks to track your progress. You're looking for a couple of things to happen. You should find that you can complete the mile in a faster time and/or your heart rate should be lower when you are done. Both of these things (faster time, lower heart rate) mean that your aerobic fitness level has improved. If your time does not improve but your heart rate is lower, that still indicates that your fitness level improved: You completed the same amount of work with less effort. Similarly, if you walk or jog the mile in a faster time at the same heart rate as before, that also demonstrates a marked improvement: You accomplished more work with the same effort as before.

SCORING CHART: WOMEN

Age	Heart Rate	Low Fitness	Moderate Fitness	High Fitness
20–29	110	>20:57	19:08–20:57	< 19:08
	120	>20:27	18:38–20:27	< 18:38
	130	>20:00	18:12–20:00	< 18:12
	140	>19:30	17:42–19:30	< 17:42
	150	>19:00	17:12–19:00	< 17:12
	160	>18:30	16:42–18:30	< 16:42
	170	>18:00	16:12–18:00	< 16:12
30–39	110	>19:46	17:52–19:46	< 17:52
	120	>19:18	17:24–19:18	< 17:24
	130	>18:48	16:54–18:48	< 16:54
	140	>18:18	16:24–18:18	< 16:24
	150	>17:48	15:54–17:48	< 15:54
	160	>17:18	15:24–17:18	< 15:24
	170	>16:54	14:55–16:54	< 14:55
40–49	110	>19:15	17:20–19:15	< 17:20
	120	>18:45	16:50–18:45	< 16:50
	130	>18:18	16:24–18:18	< 16:24
	140	>17:48	15:54–17:48	< 15:54
	150	>17:18	15:24–17:18	< 15:24
	160	>16:48	14:54–16:48	< 14:54
	170	>16:18	14:25–16:18	< 14:25
50–59	110	>18:40	17:04–18:40	< 17:04
	120	>18:12	16:36–18:12	< 16:36
	130	>17:42	16:06–17:42	< 16:06
	140	>17:18	15:36–17:18	< 15:36
	150	>16:48	15:06–16:48	< 15:06
	160	>16:18	14:36–16:18	< 14:36
	170	>15:48	14:06–15:48	< 14:06
60+	110	>18:00	16:36–18:00	< 16:36
	120	>17:30	16:06–17:30	< 16:06
	130	>17:01	15:37–17:01	< 15:37
	140	>16:31	15:09–16:31	< 15:09
	150	>16:02	14:39–16:02	< 14:39
	160	>15:32	14:12–15:32	< 14:12
	170	>15:04	13:42–15:04	< 13:42

Source: The American Heart Association

SCORING CHART: MEN

Age	Heart Rate	Low Fitness	Moderate Fitness	High Fitness
20–29	110	>19:36	17:06–19:36	<17:06
	120	>19:10	16:36–19:10	<16:36
	130	>18:35	16:06–18:35	<16:06
	140	>18:06	15:36–18:06	<15:36
	150	>17:36	15:10–17:36	<15:10
	160	>17:09	14:42–17:09	<14:42
	170	>16:39	14:12–16:39	<14:12
30–39	110	>18:21	15:54–18:21	<15:54
	120	>17:52	15:24–17:52	<15:24
	130	>17:22	14:54–17:22	<14:54
	140	>16:54	14:30–16:54	<14:30
	150	>16:26	14:00–16:26	<14:00
	160	>15:58	13:30–15:58	<13:30
	170	>15:28	13:01–15:28	<13:01
40–49	110	>18:05	15:38–18:05	<15:38
	120	>17:36	15:09–17:36	<15:09
	130	>17:07	14:41–17:07	<14:41
	140	>16:38	14:12–16:38	<14:12
	150	>16:09	13:42–16:09	<13:42
	160	>15:42	13:15–15:42	<13:15
	170	>15:12	12:45–15:12	<12:45
50–59	110	>17:49	15:22–17:49	<15:22
	120	>17:20	14:53–17:20	<14:53
	130	>16:51	14:24–16:51	<14:24
	140	>16:22	13:51–16:22	<13:51
	150	>15:53	13:26–15:53	<13:26
	160	>15:26	12:59–15:26	<12:59
	170	>14:56	12:30–14:56	<12:30
60+	110	>17:55	15:33–17:55	<15:33
	120	>17:24	15:04–17:24	<15:04
	130	>16:57	14:36–16:57	<14:36
	140	>16:28	14:07–16:28	<14:07
	150	>15:59	13:39–15:59	<13:39
	160	>15:30	13:10–15:30	<13:10
	170	>15:04	12:42–15:04	<12:42

Source: The American Heart Association

Part 3: Your Lifestyle and Attitude

Your success at any fitness program depends a great deal on your lifestyle and attitudes. Everything you do from day to day is part of your lifestyle. And your lifestyle affects your Naked Fitness. Carelessness in any area of your lifestyle can lead to serious problems. That's why it's important to know whether your lifestyle is contributing to health or illness.

Answer each question below and calculate your score using the read-the-score analysis at the end of this part to see what changes you might need to make in your lifestyle.

1. How often do you work out?
a. Four or more times weekly.
b. Three times weekly.
c. Sporadically.
d. Seldom.

2. How many hours a day do you watch television? (Working out to television exercise shows is a good habit and doesn't count toward TV-watching time.)
a. None to one.
b. One to two.
c. Two to four.
d. Four or more.

3. Are you overweight?
a. No.
b. Yes, about 5 pounds.
c. Yes, about 6 to 19 pounds.
d. Yes, 20 pounds or more.

4. **How many alcoholic drinks (beer, wine, or liquor) do you average per week?**

a. None.

b. One to seven.

c. Eight to fifteen.

d. Sixteen or more.

5. **How many cigarettes do you smoke per day?**

a. None.

b. Less than five.

c. Five to ten.

d. Ten or more.

6. **Do you smoke marijuana or use any illegal drugs?**

a. No.

b. Rarely.

c. Occasionally.

d. Frequently.

7. **Do you skip meals or eat fewer than three meals a day?**

a. Almost never.

b. Seldom.

c. Occasionally.

d. Frequently.

8. **How often do you eat fresh fruits and vegetables?**

a. Five to nine servings a day.

b. About four servings a day.

c. One to three servings a day.

d. I rarely eat fruit or vegetables.

9. **Do you eat sweets daily (sodas, sugar, cake, cookies, candy, and so forth)?**

a. Almost never.

b. Seldom.

c. Occasionally.

d. Frequently.

10. Do you get enough satisfying sleep?

a. Always.

b. Usually.

c. Occasionally.

d. Seldom.

11. How often do you feel depressed or pessimistic?

a. Almost never.

b. Seldom.

c. Occasionally.

d. Frequently.

12. Does stress or anxiety interfere with your daily activities?

a. Almost never.

b. Seldom.

c. Occasionally.

d. Frequently.

13. How often do you do something nice for yourself?

a. Almost every day.

b. Occasionally.

c. Seldom.

d. Almost never.

14. How would you describe your feelings toward your body?

a. I like to look at myself naked in a full-length mirror.

b. I occasionally look at my body in the mirror.

c. I rarely look at my body in the mirror and feel conspicuous when wearing a bathing suit in public.

d. I dislike the way I look and go to great lengths not to look at myself in the mirror.

MEDICAL READINESS FOR EXERCISE

Before you begin an exercise program, take a fitness test, or substantially increase your level of activity, make sure to answer the following questions. Developed and used by the American College of Sports Medicine, this physical activity readiness questionnaire (PAR-Q) will help determine your suitability for beginning an exercise routine or program.

- Has your doctor ever said that you have a heart condition or that you should participate in physical activity only as recommended by a doctor?
- Do you feel pain in your chest during physical activity?
- In the past month, have you had chest pain when you were not doing physical activity?
- Do you lose your balance because of dizziness? Do you ever lose consciousness?
- Do you have a bone or joint problem that could be made worse by a change in your physical activity?
- Is your doctor currently prescribing drugs for your blood pressure or a heart condition?
- Do you know of any reason you should not participate in physical activity?

15. How often do you dress in a manner that conceals your true weight?
a. Never; I like dressing to show off my physique.
b. Sometimes.
c. Occasionally.
d. As much as possible.

SCORING FOR PART 3

Give yourself a point for each "a" answer, two points for each "b" answer, three points for each "c" answer, and four points for each "d" answer.

MEDICAL READINESS FOR EXERCISE (continued)

IF YOU ANSWERED YES

If you answered yes to one or more questions, are older than age 40, and have been inactive or are concerned about your health, consult a physician before taking a fitness test or substantially increasing your physical activity. You should ask for a medical clearance along with information about specific exercise limitations you may have. In most cases, you will still be able to do any type of activity you want as long as you adhere to some guidelines.

IF YOU ANSWERED NO

If you answered no to all the PAR-Q questions, you can be reasonably sure that you can exercise safely and have a low risk of having any medical complications from exercise. It is still important to start slowly and increase gradually.

When to Delay Starting an Exercise Program

- If you are not feeling well because of a temporary illness such as a cold or a fever, wait until you feel better to begin exercising.

- If you are or may be pregnant, talk with your doctor before you become more active.

Analysis

- If you scored 15 to 24, you have an excellent lifestyle based on healthy habits, a good awareness of personal health, and an appreciation of your body.
- If you scored 25 to 34, you have a very good lifestyle, and with a little improvement, you can move into the excellent category.
- A score of 35 to 44 means you need a bit more determination and commitment to achieve a healthier lifestyle.
- If you scored 45 to 54, you may be taking unnecessary risks with your health, and you should set a goal to improve those areas in which you scored high.

- A score of 55 or more indicates that you may be ignoring good health habits. You might be in a danger zone and should seriously think about making important lifestyle changes. Naked Fitness will help you.

I recommend taking the Naked Fitness assessment test every six weeks. Seeing improvements can be a good motivator to continue exercising. If you follow my program to a tee, you'll see noticeable improvement in your scores and feel energized and confident about your physical abilities.

PART 2

The Naked Fitness Workout

4

THE NAKED FITNESS
EXERCISES

Many of my clients (athletes in particular) are convinced that exercise has to be painful to be beneficial. Exercising should never be painful, so ignore the overworked fitness anthem, "No pain, no gain." Instead, think of Naked Fitness exercises as "all gain, no pain."

My Naked Fitness exercises are gentle. But this doesn't mean they aren't intense. They are. You work a lot of muscles in a short amount of time. And you'll see a significant improvement in muscle tone and shape, strength, posture, and energy, with the added bonus of a healthier heart and increased metabolism.

The Naked Fitness exercises emphasize a balance between strength and flexibility, endurance, and the development of self-awareness. And you absolutely will get results and be thrilled by the benefits described below.

POSTURE. One of people's most revealing characteristics is the way they carry themselves. Confidence emanates from people who hold their head and chest high and their shoulders back. Think about it: How much strength and conviction emanates from a person who walks and sits with rounded shoulders and a hunched back?

As I've emphasized, an important focus of these exercises is alignment and balance of the body—in other words, posture. Since many of us spend a large part of our lives with poor posture—hunched over a computer keyboard, a steering wheel, or our kitchen counter—we need exercises to correct this imbalance and improve the way we look and feel. These exercises will accomplish that.

STRENGTH AND TONE. My exercises develop lean muscle, which is "metabolically active." This means your muscles burn body fat more efficiently than fat tissue or untoned muscle, even at rest. Blood circulation to fatty areas of the body is often sluggish. Consequently, fat is more difficult to metabolize in those spots. Exercise to the rescue! Exercise increases circulation in fat storage areas and thus helps pry loose stubborn fat. The Naked Fitness exercises also firm your muscles to help hold any residual body fat in place better so that it jiggles less. And they help iron out those dimply pockets of fat known as cellulite, thus improving overall skin tone. All of these wonderful outcomes delay the signs of aging so you'll look great naked, no matter what your age.

FUNCTIONAL FITNESS. This term describes exercises that strengthen multiple muscles on multiple planes, mimicking how we use them in real life (hence the functional aspect). Functional fitness does more than strengthen: It improves your coordination and balance, prevents strength imbalances, and targets the stabilizing muscles that you call on throughout the day. Simple things such as tying your shoes or putting on hosiery will no longer leave you breathless. And you'll be able to walk upstairs and still talk when you get to the top.

INJURY PREVENTION. My exercises strengthen your tendons and ligaments. Your musculoskeletal system thus adapts to tolerate more stress with less chance of injury. You'll be more apt to avoid orthopedic problems such as shoulder impingement, back pain, and neck pain.

EMOTIONAL WELL-BEING. These exercises have a positive influence on your emotional well-being and body image. Because of their gentle moves, they may also be the answer to help you find peace with yourself and your place in the world. Expect to get a physical workout and spiritual practice at the same time.

Minimal Equipment Required

Another benefit of my Naked Fitness exercises is that they require little equipment. And what you do need is very inexpensive. Here's a rundown.

AN EXERCISE MAT. You'll need a lightweight mat that rolls up easily to provide support and comfort for floor exercises. A mat will also help cushion your knees. (A folded blanket also works in a pinch for floor exercises.)

RESISTANCE TUBING. First employed as a rehab device by doctors in the 1960s, resistance tubing has seen an explosive growth in popularity among exercisers in the past few years. In addition to its convenience (you don't have to stash it under the bed or in the closet like the latest devices being hawked on infomercials), they provide smooth resistance throughout a full range of motion, and they increase intensity by offering the training benefits of continuous tension. This develops nice, balanced muscles and is easy on the joints.

Tubing usually comes in several progressive levels of resistance: light, medium, and heavy, designated by the color of the tubing. Most of my exercises use medium-resistance tubing. Tubing ranges anywhere from $6 to $20, depending on how many you get and where you buy them, which is nice if you're a budget-conscious exerciser.

LIGHT DUMBBELLS (3 TO 8 POUNDS). Dumbbells—also known as free weights—are excellent for firming up muscle and building strength in the shortest possible time. Exercises with dumbbells work groups of muscles and do an excellent job of building overall strength and muscle tone. They also isolate and define specific muscles.

STABILITY BALL. Exercising on a stability ball has lots of benefits, such as increased muscle tone and flexibility, improved posture and coordination, and greater body awareness. With a stability ball, your muscles work hard to keep you balanced. Balance work strengthens your abs and back, so you reduce your risk of injury. You'll see a difference not only in how your clothes fit but in how you feel—stronger, better coordinated, and more confident.

SOFT BALL. In a sporting-goods store, look for a spongy, soft, lightweight ball about the size of a softball. You'll use a ball like this in several of my exercises.

Most of the Naked Fitness exercises force you to move your own body weight without any equipment at all. Body weight exercises provide an amazing workout because you must stay balanced and stable as you do them. Performing exercises in which you move your own body weight helps you in other activities too, such as biking and various sports. Any exercise you do with your own body weight is beneficial and functional—the perfect way to keep your muscles toned, strong, and balanced.

For more information on this equipment, visit www.nakedfitness.com.

Naked Fitness Exercise Guidelines

To understand how the Naked Fitness exercises work, read through the exercise descriptions first. Pay attention to the letters A, B, C, or D after each exercise. These correspond to your fitness test results. If those results indicate that you will do the A routine and A exercises, focus on those exercises and try them one by one. Expect to feel awkward at first; that is normal. Just remember that each move is designed to motivate, shape, relax, and inspire.

Here are some important guidelines:

• Focus on proper form and technique. Don't just go through the motions. Fast, jerky repetitions don't isolate muscles but instead place harmful stress on the joints, ligaments, and tendons. Not only is this an unproductive way to tone muscles, but it's also a dangerous exercise habit to adopt because it increases your risk of injury. Incorrect form reduces stress on the muscles and bones and can lead to injury.

- Be careful to move only the joints and body parts specified for each exercise.

- For many of the standing exercises, distribute your weight equally on both legs. This will keep you from losing your balance and possibly injuring yourself. Also, bend your knees slightly to protect your lower back.

- To get the most from every repetition, move through a complete range of motion. Range of motion is the full path of an exercise, from extension to contraction and back again.

- Breathe properly. With every repetition, inhale just before the lift and exhale as you complete it. Try to synchronize inhalation and exhalation rhythmically with the motion of the rep. Never hold your breath. Holding your breath cuts the oxygen supply to the blood and, coupled with the exertion of the lift, could cause lightheadedness or fainting.

- Know your limits. Overdoing can lead to strains, a condition characterized by swelling and pain in the muscles, and pulls, which are acute tears of muscle fibers. While you're exercising, pay attention whenever your body sends you a pain message. This is a warning, just like a yellow traffic light. The pain message doesn't mean you have hurt yourself; however, if you push the exercise beyond this point—into the continually painful red zone—you may risk hurting yourself and slowing your progress. Perform the exercises all the way through the pain-free green zone and up to the yellow light. Don't exercise into the red zone. You're honoring your body by doing only as much as feels comfortable.

- Never train a sore body part. If you find that a muscle group is still sore from the previous workout, don't train it.

- Stay hydrated by drinking plenty of water. Drink a cup (8 ounces) of water before and after exercise, as well as every 15 minutes during exercise.

The exercises are divided into stretches and strengthening moves. Remember, after the name of the stretch or strengthening move, I've noted which exercises are used in the A (upper-back), B (mid-back), C (low-back), and D (total posture and body) routines. I cover these routines in the next chapter.

Naked Fitness Stretches

CHIN CHEST STRETCH (A)

Begin in a seated or standing position. Keep your shoulders down and squeeze your shoulder blades together. Hold your head aligned over the top of your spine (neutral position). Inhale.

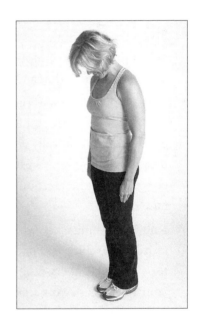

Exhale. Slowly drop your chin toward your chest. Hold in this position for two to three counts.

Inhale. Lift your chin and return to the neutral position.

Repeat two to three times.

TIP: For a deeper stretch, place a soft ball, a pair of socks, or a rolled-up towel under your chin and press into the object on the stretch. The object should be large enough to hold in place with your head in neutral position.

SIDE NECK STRETCH (A, B, and D)

Begin in a seated or standing position. Keep your shoulders down and squeeze your shoulder blades together. Hold your head aligned over the top of your spine (neutral position). Inhale.

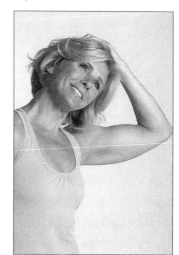

Exhale. Slowly drop your ear toward your right shoulder and use your left hand to assist the stretch.

Hold in this position for two to three counts.

Inhale. Lift your chin and return to the neutral position.

Repeat on the opposite side

Repeat two to three times.

TIP: For a deeper stretch, place a soft ball, a pair of socks, or a rolled-up towel under your chin.

TILTED NECK STRETCH UP (A)

Begin in a seated or standing position. Keep your shoulders down and squeeze your shoulder blades together. Hold your head aligned over the top of your spine (neutral position). Inhale.

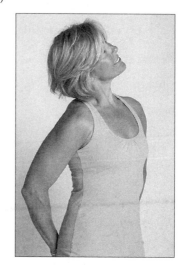

Exhale. Slowly drop your ear toward one shoulder. Then turn your chin toward the ceiling.

Hold in this position for two to three counts.

Inhale. Lift your chin and return to the neutral position.

Repeat on the opposite side

Repeat two to three times.

TIP: For a deeper stretch, place a soft ball, a pair of socks, or a rolled-up towel under your chin.

TILTED NECK STRETCH DOWN (A)

Begin in a seated or standing position. Keep your
shoulders down and
squeeze your shoulder
blades together. Hold your
head aligned over the top
of your spine (neutral
position). Inhale.

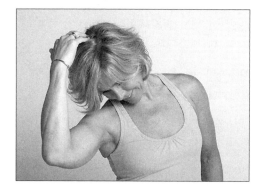

Exhale. Slowly drop your
ear toward your shoulder.
Then turn your chin toward your right armpit and
use your right hand to assist.

Hold in this position for two to three counts.

Inhale. Lift your chin and return to the neutral position.

Repeat on the opposite side.

Repeat two to three times.

TIP: For a deeper stretch, place a soft ball, a pair of socks, or a towel under your chin.

SINGLE-HAND WRIST/WALL STRETCH (A and B)

Begin in a seated or
standing position.
Reach one arm front
and press into the wall
if available. Turn your
palm downward. Keep
your shoulders down
and squeeze your shoul-
der blades together
(neutral position).
Inhale.

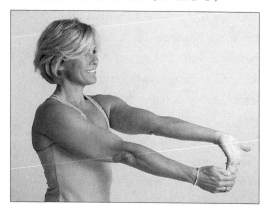

Exhale as you hold in this position for two to three counts.

Inhale and release the stretch.

Repeat two to three times. Then repeat on the opposite side.

CHIN ROTATION (A)

Begin in a seated or standing position. Keep your shoulders down
and squeeze your shoulder blades
together. Hold your head aligned
over the top of your spine (neutral
position). Inhale.

Exhale. Slowly turn your head as far
to the right as you can.

Hold in this position for two to three
counts.

Inhale. Return to the center while
keeping your chin parallel to the floor.

Repeat on the opposite side.

Repeat again on each side.

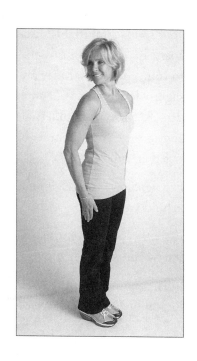

HAND BEHIND BACK NECK STRETCH (D)

This is a slight variation of the Side Neck Stretch. Begin in a standing position with your feet comfortably apart. Place one arm behind your back. Lean your ear to the opposite side and gently push the top of your head toward your shoulder. Hold this position for 10 to 12 counts. Repeat twice; then perform the exercise on the opposite side.

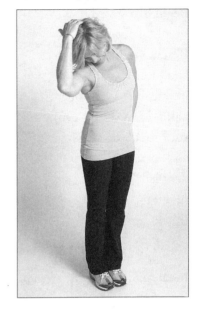

CHEST STRETCH LOW (A, B, and D)

Begin in a standing position with your feet a comfortable distance apart. Extend your arms out to your sides so that they are slightly lower than your shoulders. Keep your shoulders down and squeeze your shoulder blades together. Inhale.

Exhale. Slowly stretch your arms behind your body.

Hold this position for two to three counts.

Inhale and release the stretch. Repeat two to three times.

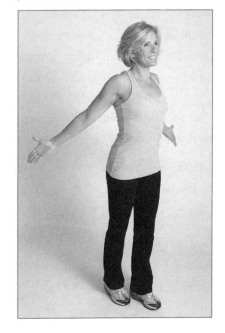

TIP: For a deeper stretch, place your hands on a door frame and press your body forward into the stretch.

CHEST STRETCH HIGH (B, C, and D)

Begin in a standing position with your feet a comfortable distance apart. Extend your arms out to your sides and bent, keeping your upper arms parallel to the floor. Keep your shoulders down and squeeze your shoulder blades together. Inhale.

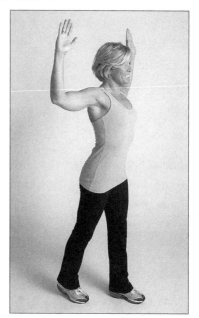

Exhale. Slowly stretch your arms behind your body.

Hold this position for two to three counts.

Inhale and release the stretch. Repeat two to three times.

TIP: For a deeper stretch, place your hands on a door frame and press your body forward into the stretch.

CROSSED ARM STRETCH (A and B)

Begin in a seated or standing position. Keep your shoulders down.
Inhale.

Exhale. Extend your right arm and
reach it across your chest. Pull your
arm with your left hand to get a good
stretch in your arm.

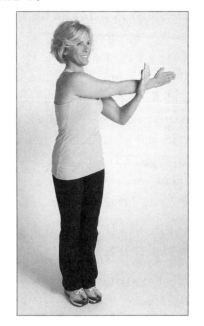

Hold this position for two to three
counts.

Inhale. Release the stretch and return
to the center. Repeat the stretch on
the opposite side.

Repeat twice on each side.

ARM ACROSS LOW (B)

Begin in a seated or standing position.

Extend your right arm across your torso
at a downward angle. Keeping your
shoulders pressed down, pull your right
arm across your body with your left
hand. Inhale.

Exhale. Hold this position for two to
three counts.

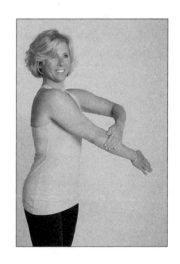

Inhale and release to the center and
repeat on the opposite side.

Repeat on both sides.

OVERHEAD TRICEPS STRETCH (A)

Begin in a seated or standing position. Reach one arm overhead and bend your elbow so that you reach toward the center of your spine. Inhale.

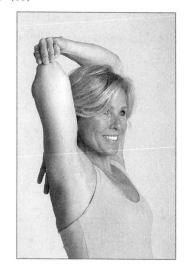

Gently assist the elbow of your stretching arm so that it reaches toward the ceiling.

Exhale. Hold this position for two to three counts.

Inhale and repeat the stretch on the opposite side.

Repeat on both sides.

FIGURE 8 ARM STRETCH (B)

Begin in a seated or standing position.

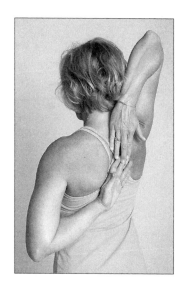

Reach your right arm behind your back to the center of your spine, with the palm facing away from your body.

Extend your left hand overhead, and then reach to the center of your upper back, with your palm toward your body. If your hands cannot connect, use a towel to assist the stretch.

Squeeze your shoulder blades together to open your chest. Inhale.

Exhale and hold two to three counts. Inhale and release the stretch.

Perform the stretch four times. Then do the stretch on the opposite side.

FORWARD ROLL DOWN (A)

Stand with your feet about shoulder-width apart. Extend your arms overhead.

Bend both knees slightly and lower your hands to your thighs. Bend with a rounded back toward your feet.

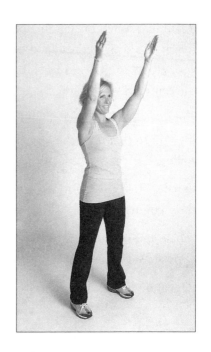

Keep your neck relaxed, hands on thighs and belly pulled into your spine to support your upper body. Exhale as you roll down and hold this position for two to three counts.

Inhale. Roll up, supporting your upper body with your hands on your legs, if needed.

Repeat three to five times.

TIP: If you have had any lower back injuries, you can walk your hands down a wall or a chair to support your spine.

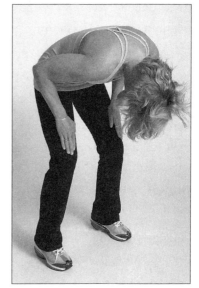

FULL SIDE BEND CIRCLE—LIVE-ILIATES™ STRETCH (D)
While standing or seated, raise your arms overhead. Inhale as you
reach to the side and bend sideways and down toward your knees and
then toward your feet. Stretch up to the other side and exhale as you
straighten your body, completing the circle to an upright posture.
Repeat 10 times, alternating sides.

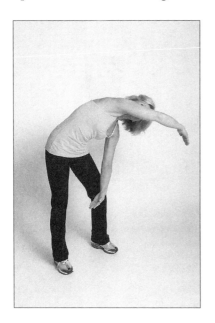
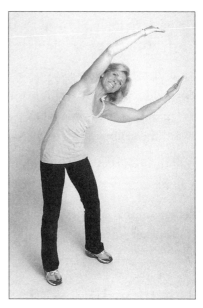

IT BAND STRETCH (C and D)

The IT band is a layer of connective tissue that runs down the outside of the leg from the outer side of your hip to below your knee, where it attaches to the outer side of your upper shin bone. When this tissue is injured, your knee may hurt. This stretch may help prevent injury.

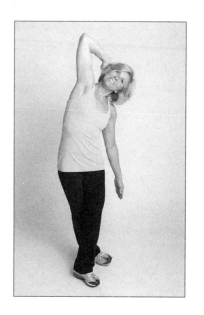

Begin in a standing position. Cross your right leg slightly behind your left leg. Reach your right elbow toward the ceiling. Lean to the side.

Hold this position for 10 counts. Then repeat.

Change sides and perform two times on the other side.

STANDING HIP FLEXOR STRETCH (C)

Begin with your feet in a "split stance," with your left foot in front and your right foot behind. Your right foot should be turned slightly inward.

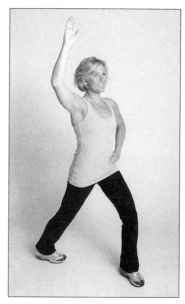

Press your hips forward to get a good stretch in the front of your hip. Hold this position for 10 counts. Repeat the stretch at least two times.

Repeat the stretch on the opposite side at least two times.

HIP FLEXOR STRETCH BALANCE (C and D)

Stand on your left leg and bring your right foot up on a bench or ball. Hold the bent knee stretch for two to three counts, leaning slightly forward if balance and flexibility permit. Return your foot to the floor and repeat. Change sides and perform the stretch two times. You may hold on to a chair for balance.

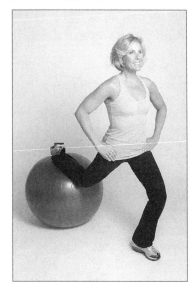

TIP: As your balance gets better, try to perform a King Dancer pose from yoga. Bend your left knee and grasp the inside of your left foot with your left hand. Bring your left foot and your right arm up toward the ceiling as you lean your torso forward. Hold for 5 to 10 breaths. Repeat on the opposite side.

SEATED FOOT CROSS (C)

Sit in a chair or on a ball. Keep your right foot on the ground. Cross your left foot over your right knee.

Lean forward at your waist and rest your hands on your bent knee for balance. Hold this position for 10 counts. Repeat the stretch twice, and then repeat on the opposite side.

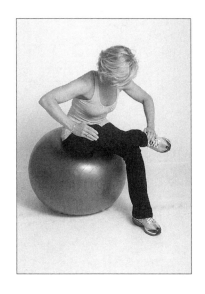

BENT KNEE SIDE STRETCH (B)

Lie on your right side on an exercise mat or other comfortable surface. Bend your knees to the side.

Inhale. With arms outstretched, extend one arm from your body and open your chest to the ceiling while reaching your hand to the side.

Exhale. Hold this position for two to three counts.

Inhale and return to the closed-hand position.

As you do this stretch, keep the movement in a straight line following your shoulders. Perform two to three times on each side.

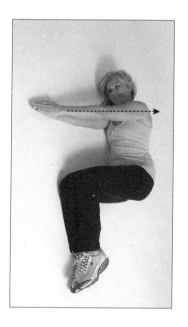 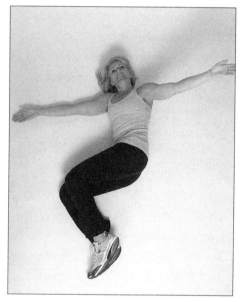

DOUBLE KNEE TO SIDE STRETCH (C)

Start on your back with both
knees bent in the air and
your arms out to the side.
Slowly lower your legs to the
side and hold 10 to 12
counts. Repeat twice on each
side.

TIP: Place your hands under
heavy weights to hold to
anchor the upper body.

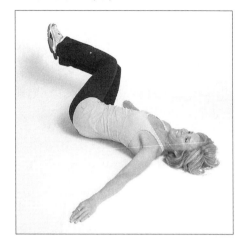

SPINE TWIST UP (B, C, and D)

Begin in a seated posi-
tion. Cross your right
heel over your knee, as
shown.

Let your left elbow rest
on the bent knee. Inhale.

Exhale. Rotate your torso
and look over your right
shoulder. Hold this posi-
tion for two to three
counts.

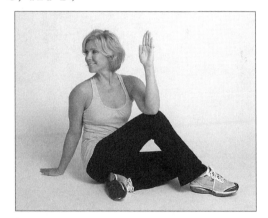

Inhale and release the stretch.

Repeat this move four times; then repeat four times on the opposite
side.

CAT TO COW (B)

Position yourself on all fours on an exercise mat or other soft surface.

Draw your chin into your chest and your belly into your spine, dropping your tailbone downward. Inhale.

Exhale. Round your spine and hold this position for two to three counts.

Inhale. Lift your chin. Press your belly toward your thighs and press your toes into the floor with your heels upward.

Repeat this move four times.

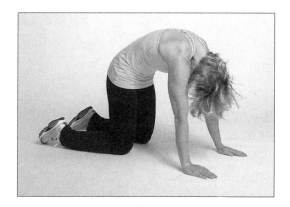

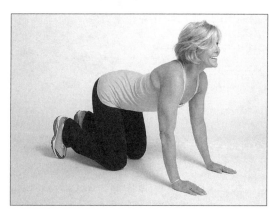

KNEE TO CHEST HIP FLEXOR STRETCH (C and D)

Lie on your back
and place a rolled
towel or yoga mat
under your hips be-
tween your tailbone
and rib cage. Draw
one knee toward
your chest and ex-
tend the other leg
straight to floor.

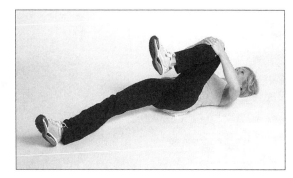

Flex the toes of your elongated leg toward the ceiling and work on getting the back of your thigh on the ground. Feel the stretch in the front
of your thigh and the back of the bent knee.

Hold for 10 to 30 seconds and repeat on the other side. Perform this
stretch two to three times on each side.

CROSS-OVER STRETCH (C AND D)

Lie on your back on
an exercise mat or
comfortable surface.
Place your left hand
behind your head.
Lift and cross your
left leg over to the
opposite side of
your body. Press
toward the floor
with your left hand.
Hold for 10 to 12
counts and repeat
twice. Repeat on
the opposite side.

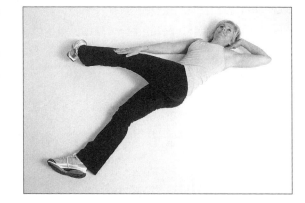

KNEE TUCK (D)

Lie on your back on an exercise mat or other comfortable surface. Bring both knees to your chest and gently hug them. Hold for 10 to 12 seconds, then release the hug. During the exercise, press your hips and tailbone down into the floor. Repeat the exercise two to three times on each side.

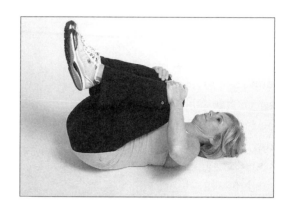

SEXY SPINE (C)

Lie on your back on an exercise mat or comfortable surface. Place your left hand behind your head. Bend your left knee. Bring your knee toward your chest and then across the body. Press your knee toward the floor. Keep your shoulder blades on the floor. Hold for 10 to 12 counts and repeat twice. Repeat on the opposite side.

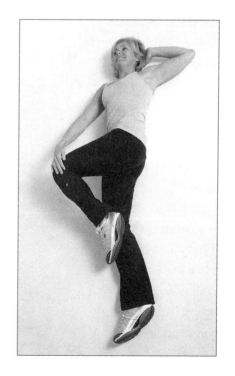

Strengthening Moves

ARM CIRCLE HANGS (A)

Stand with your feet comfortably apart. Grasp a light dumbbell (3 to 8 pounds) in one hand.

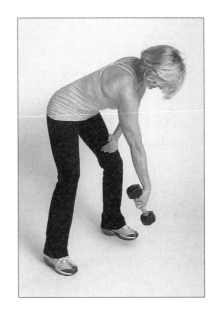

Extend one arm down and slowly circle your hand in a clockwise direction eight times. Then circle again in a counterclockwise direction eight times.

Repeat on other side.

CHIN TILTS (A)

Lie on your back on an exercise mat or other comfortable surface. Point your chin toward the ceiling.

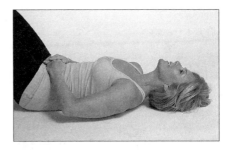

Then slowly press your chin toward your chest, lengthening the back of your neck.

Hold this position for two to three counts.

Release and repeat 8 to 12 times.

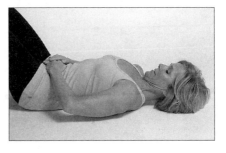

WALL LEANS (A)

Stand with your back to the wall. Your heels should be twelve to eighteen inches from the wall.

Place a rolled-up towel at the top back of your head and press your head to the wall.

Inhale. Lift your chest off the wall, keeping your body in a straight line. This will resemble a board leaning against a wall. Support your body with weight anchored in feet and head against wall.

Hold this position for two to three counts, and then rest your body back up against the wall.

Repeat 8 to 12 times.

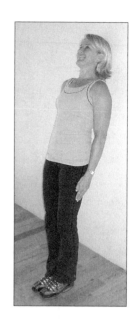

TIP: If you have had any type of neck or back injury, please perform head floor leans (below) instead until you can work your way up to a standing position.

HEAD FLOOR LEANS (A)

Lie on your back on an exercise mat or other comfortable surface. Keep your neck in a neutral position (parallel to the floor) with a small folded towel placed under your neck.

Inhale. Press your buttocks against the floor. Exhale. While maintaining a neutral spine, lift your rib cage and shoulder blades off the floor

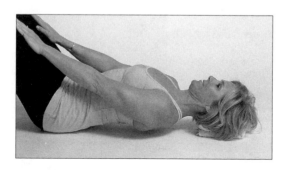

about one inch. Hold this position for two to three counts. Your body is supported by the back of your head and hips.

Inhale and lower your upper back to the floor.

Repeat 8 to 12 times.

SHOULDER BLADE SQUEEZE (A, B, and D)

Stand with your feet a comfortable distance apart. Raise your arms out to your sides so that they are at shoulder-height and bent at the elbows.

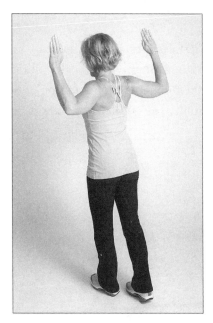

Keep your shoulders down and squeeze your shoulder blades together. Inhale.

Exhale. Slowly open your arms behind your body.

Hold this position for two to three counts.

Inhale and release. Repeat three to five times.

TIP: For a deeper stretch, place your hands in a door frame and press your body forward into the stretch.

SHOULDER BLADE SQUEEZE WITH ROW (B and D)
Stand with your feet a comfortable distance apart. Grasp one light
dumbbell. Bend at the hips so that your torso is parallel to the floor.
Keep your knees slightly bent.

Squeeze your shoulder blades together; then pull one hand up toward
your rib cage. Squeeze at the top of the move and hold for two to three
counts. Slowly lower the weight toward the floor. Inhale on the lowering phase and exhale on the pull.

Perform 8 to 12 repetitions on each side. You can also use resistance
tubing. Simply anchor the tubing with your feet placed in the center of
the tubing. From a standing position, pull the tubing straight up to just
under your underarms. Lower slowly and repeat.

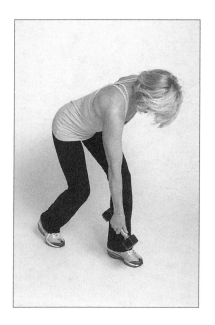
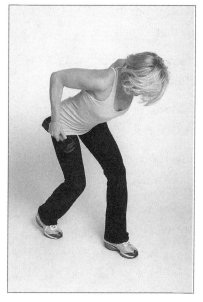

WIDE PULLS (A, B, and D)

Standing or seated, hold resistance tubing at shoulder height with hands in front of elbows. Keep your shoulders down and squeeze your shoulder blades together. Inhale.

Exhale. Slowly open your arms and stretch the tubing across your chest.

Hold this position for two to three counts.

Inhale and release. Perform 8 to 12 reps.

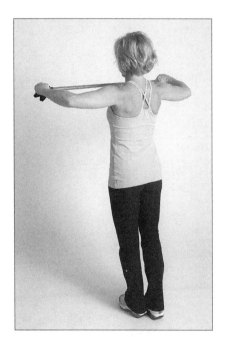

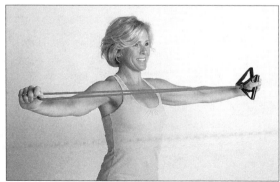

ROTATOR CUFF UP (A and B)

Step with one foot on medium-resistance tubing to secure it.

Bend your elbow to a 90-degree angle, with your hand facing front and your elbow close to your body.

Slowly rotate your hand toward the middle of your body.

Return to starting position.

Repeat 8 to 12 times on each side.

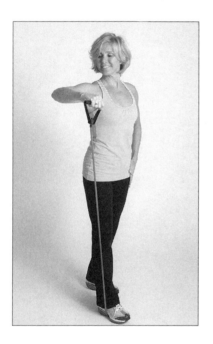

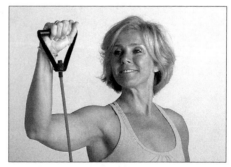

ROTATOR CUFF SIDE (A and B)

Start with light- to medium-resistance tubing. Hold the tubing in your right hand at your hip keeping tension on the tubing.

With your left arm bent close to your ribs, rotate your hand outward to the side and hold for two to three counts.

Keep your shoulders relaxed and your forearm parallel to the ground.

Repeat 8 to 12 times on each side.

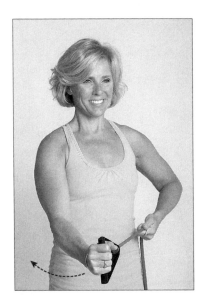

TOWEL TWIST OUTS (A)

Stand with your feet a comfortable distance apart. Hold a towel or resistance tubing down across your thighs. Press your arms outward, squeezing your shoulders and rotating your thumbs to the outside. Hold this position for two to three counts. Keep your shoulders relaxed and press down throughout the move.

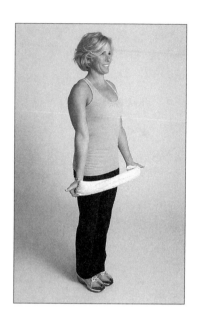

Slowly return to the starting position.

Perform 8 to 12 repetitions.

SINGLE-ARM WIDE PULL, THUMBS UP (A)

Stand with your feet a comfortable distance apart. Hold a towel or resistance tubing at chest height. Stretch your arms out in front of you so that they are parallel to the floor. Your thumb on the side that you will be exercising should be pointing upward.

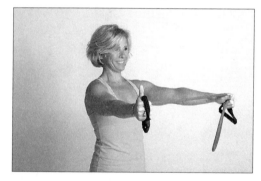

Keeping your arms extended and straight, move one arm out to the outside. Hold this position for two to three counts while keeping the

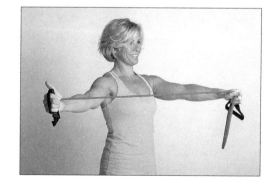

other arm stable. Keep your shoulders relaxed and press down throughout the move.

Slowly return your arms to the center and repeat the move on the opposite arm.

Perform 8 to 12 repetitions.

SINGLE-ARM WIDE PULL, PALMS DOWN (A)

Stand with your feet a comfortable distance apart. Hold a resistance tubing at chest height. Stretch your arms out in front of you so that they are parallel to the floor. Your palm on the side that you will be exercising should be facing down.

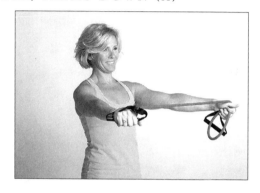

Keeping your arms extended and straight, move one arm out to the outside. Hold this position for two to three counts while keeping the other arm stable. Keep your shoulders relaxed and press down throughout the move.

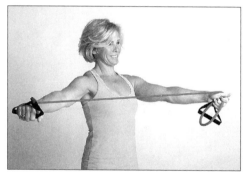

Slowly return your arms to the center and repeat the move on the opposite arm.

Perform 8 to 12 repetitions.

SINGLE-ARM LAT PULL DOWN (B)

Begin in a seated or standing position. Practice good posture, with your spine aligned, your shoulders back, and head up. Grasp a resistance band at each end and raise your arms above your head. Keep your hands a little further than shoulder-width apart. Adjust your grip so that there is no slack in the band at this resting position. The band should be taut, but not fully stretched out. The closer the hands are to one another when grasping the band, the harder the exercise will be.

Pull one arm down, allowing your elbow to squeeze into your side. Return your arm back up over your head to the starting position.

Repeat the movement 15 times on each side.

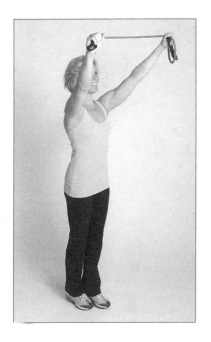
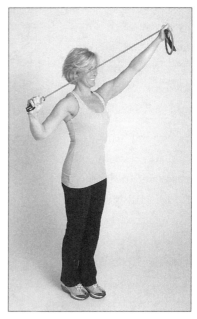

SHOULDER ARM CIRCLES (B)

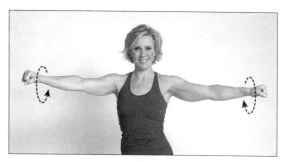

You may use a 3- to 8-pound dumbbell in each hand, or use an empty gallon of milk filled with water to add resistance.

Lift your arms out to your sides. Circle your arms 10 times toward the front, and 10 times toward the back.

SIDE LUNGE (C and D)

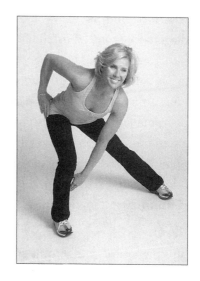

Stand with your feet together. Step to the right side, bending your right knee to transfer your weight to your right foot. Reach your left hand to your right knee and keep your toes pointed forward and weight on the heels on the lunge.

Push back to the center and perform the movement on the left side. Continue alternating from side to side for a total of 20 lunges.

TIP: Add a dumbbell and touch the weight to the floor on the lunge part of the movement to make the exercise more challenging.

CURTSY (C)

Stand with your feet shoulder-width apart. Step back with your right foot, bending your right leg behind the left in a "curtsy" position. Reach your right hand toward your foot. Pause and then bring your right foot back to starting position. Step your left foot behind your right and continue alternating sides for 20 repetitions. Stand up between each curtsy.

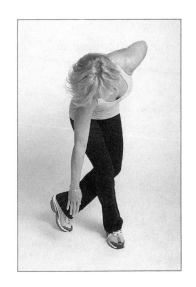

CORNER MINI-LUNGE (C)

Stand with your feet together and your toes pointing forward. Step diagonally about 12 to 20 inches into a small lunge, keeping your knees bent. Bend slightly from your hips. Touch the floor (as if picking up a small object) and push back to a standing position. Step with the opposite foot diagonally to the other side and return to standing. Perform 20 alternating lunges.

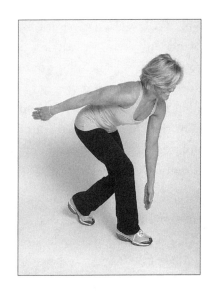

TIP: Use small steps and keep your hips high until you become strong enough to touch the floor.

SIDE PLANK ON KNEE (B and D)

Start on your side with your elbow under your shoulders. Bend both knees. Inhale to prepare and exhale while lifting hips off the ground. Hold two to three counts and return to the floor. Perform 8 to 12 repetitions.

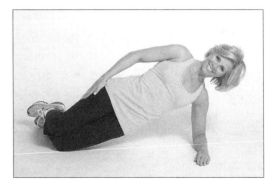

TIP: An advanced version is to hold each lift 10 to 30 counts and perform 3 to 5 repetitions or extend your legs.

KNEES BENT, ARMS REACH ACROSS (B)

Start on your back with both knees bent to your left side. Arms are wide on the floor, with your chest facing the ceiling. Reach your right hand across your chest to your left arm; then return to the starting open position. Perform five to eight times on both sides.

TIP: Try to keep your hips and knees stable on the floor.

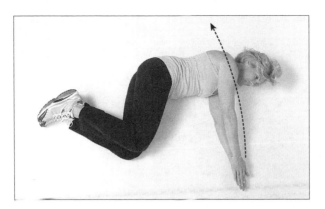

RAINBOW REACHES (B)

Lie on your back with both knees bent to the left side. Arms are wide on the floor, with your chest facing the ceiling. Reach your right hand up and over your head in an arc to your left side and back to starting open position. Reach over and around five to eight times. Bring knees to your other side and perform five to eight repetitions.

TIP: Try to keep your hips and knees stable on the floor.

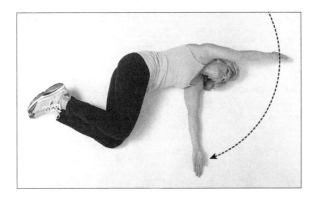

BRIDGE (C and D)

Lie on the floor with your knees bent and your arms at your sides. Inhale to prepare and exhale as you lift your hips toward the ceiling. Keep your rib cage low and squeeze the backs of your thighs at the top of the lift for two to three counts.

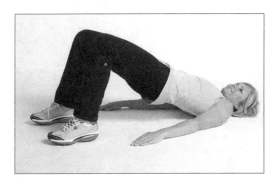

Lower to the floor as you inhale and tap the ground with your back-side. Perform 15 to 20 repetitions.

TIP: As you become stronger, add a ball under your feet and lift your hips or add a small, soft ball between your knees to strengthen your inner thighs.

BRIDGE WITH LEG LIFTS (C and D)

Lie on the floor with your knees bent and your arms at your sides. Inhale to prepare and exhale as you lift your hips toward the ceiling. Keep your rib cage low and squeeze the backs of your thighs at the top. Hold your hips in place and alternate lifting your feet slightly off the floor while maintaining hips parallel to the ground. Perform 20 alternating lifts.

TIP: As you become stronger balance your feet on a step or ball while alternating foot lifts.

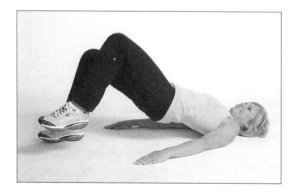

PELVIC TILT (C and D)

Lie on the floor with your knees bent. Keep some space between the floor and the small of your back (this is a neutral spine position).

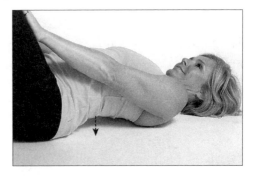

Inhale to prepare. Exhale, press your lower back into the floor, and tilt your pelvis toward your rib cage. Press your lower back down and pull in your belly. Hold for two to three counts. Return to the neutral spine position.

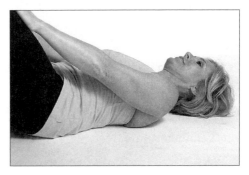

Perform 10 to 15 pelvic tilts.

HAMSTRING CURL (C)

Lie on the floor with your legs straight on top of a stability ball and your arms at your sides. Inhale and raise your hips up off the floor. Exhale as you roll the ball in toward your hips. Then return to the

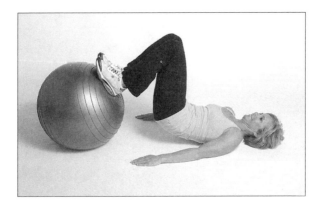

legs-extended position. Lower your hips and repeat. Perform 10 to 15 repetitions.

TIP: As you become stronger, keep your hips lifted between ball rolls.

TOE PULLS (C)

Lie on the floor with your legs extended up against a wall or in the air. Keep your feet parallel to the ceiling and flex your toes toward your shins. Do not point your toes or feet in this exercise but keep them relaxed between each flex. Move your toes downward. Perform 10 repetitions in three positions: Feet together, toes apart, and heels apart.

TIP: If it is too difficult to place your feet at a 90-degree angle, increase the distance from the wall by about 45 degrees.

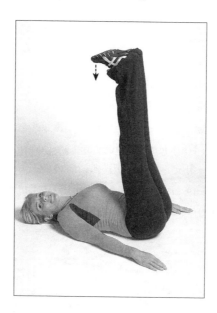

SWIMMER (C and D)

Lie face down with your arms and legs extended. Lift your right hand and left foot slightly above the ground. Switch to lift your left hand and right foot. Alternate lifts for 20 repetitions.

TIP: Keep your head in a neutral position with your chin tucked slightly down. and your neck in a straight line with your back.

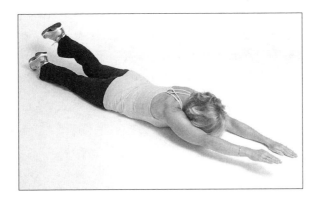

POINTER (C and D)

Start on your hands and knees. Balance your weight firmly on all points. Next, reach your left arm forward and your right leg back in a parallel line to the floor. Hold this position for three to five counts. Return to the starting position and perform on the other side. Alternate movements for 10 repetitions.

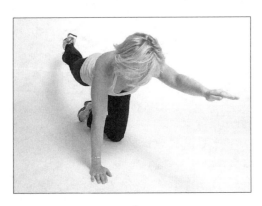

SUPERMAN (B and D)

Lie face down on the floor with your arms and legs extended. Pull your belly into your spine. Lift your arms and legs slightly from the floor. Hold two to three counts and return to rest. Perform 8 to 12 repetitions.

TIP: Do not lift your chin, but rather keep your head in a straight line with your spine (this is the neutral position). More is not better with this movement. Keep your lifts low to the ground and your body extended.

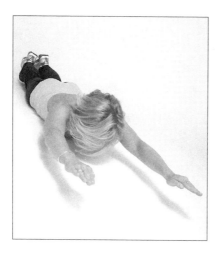

Now that you've oriented yourself to my Naked Fitness exercises, let's move on to the routines.

5

THE NAKED FITNESS PERSONALIZED ROUTINES

More than 25 years ago, I walked into a racquet sports club with my high-top exercise shoes, pink leg warmers, twisted terry cloth headband, and belted thong leotard. I had cassette tapes in hand and cue cards in place. This was my first aerobics class as an instructor. Popular uptempo hits played through the studio as we bounced, stretched, and kicked our way through the workout on linoleum-covered concrete floors. So much has changed since that first class—certifications, step and spinning classes, yoga, Pilates, foam rollers, and BOSU balls. And, thankfully, that thong leotard is now long gone.

My focus in recent years has been on showing people how to look better and live better with simple, gentle moves that allow them to get lean and serene in the shortest time possible. My easy-to-do-at-home workouts combine ease of movement and structural integrity for tall posture, graceful movements, and the ability to get out of bed each morning without feeling like the Tin Man in search of his oil can.

It took me many years to refine my method. I attended seminars, studied fat loss, and began experimenting with different kinds of workouts. To my satisfaction, what came to be called Naked Fitness worked and didn't require hours and hours of commitment.

Because I'm a fitness trainer, you'd think I'd be religious about working out, at least 60 minutes, every day, seven days a week. And I am . . . sometimes. But every so often, life becomes overwhelming (I have three teenagers, travel a lot, and run a business), and some days I just can't find the time to exercise. Sound familiar?

People want results, but they don't want to spend a lot of time working out. That's what the Naked Fitness routines deliver. They usually only take around 15 minutes! That's right: Run through the workout once, and you're done. However, don't think the workout is easy. You do have to adhere to the pacing of the workout, resting only as long as it takes to move to your next exercise, or else it won't be as effective. You're going to work important areas of your body very quickly, and your heart rate will soar.

A growing body of research shows that short workouts, as long as you put the same energy into them, are just as beneficial to your health in the long term as longer ones. The latest findings even show that the benefits from these workouts last over decades and that with relatively small amounts of exercise that people can easily fit into their daily lives, they can improve their health, fitness, and well-being.

So if you're tired of trying to spend hours getting a buff body, you'll love my shorter, kinder, gentler (but extremely effective) approach that promises major results—fast.

My brand of personal training has always been a very individualized one, which is why these workouts are customized to the area of your body that needs the most attention; hence the A, B, C, and D workouts. So you'll want to pull out the results of your fitness test and see which workout you should perform.

With the Naked Fitness workouts, you will concentrate on specific areas, with focused, selective exercises organized into a specially designed routine, to get your body in great shape.

Each efficient 15-minute workout targets key muscle groups with fluid exercise moves. The slow, controlled movements train muscles to work in patterns that mimic the motions of real life and build strength, flexibility, and muscle balance simultaneously. Your body isn't the only winner; since this workout summons your full concentration, it's also a great stress melter.

Get Mentally Ready

Starting a new routine or getting back into working out can be daunting. We cringe when we see ourselves stuffed into our stretchy workout clothes or shorts. And it's tough to face the long road back to where we left off the last time we tried to get in shape. But I feel that the best way to get motivated is to put those big impediments out of your mind and focus on one small step at a time. Here are some suggestions to help you get in the right frame of mind:

- Sit down in a quiet place. Close your eyes and try to remember how great you used to feel when you were working out—from the endorphin highs to how the fat started melting right off.

- Organize your schedule as best you can to accommodate your 15-minute workout. Setting a regular time and place for exercise is not necessarily a must. But, make sure you plan it into your schedule and pencil it into your weekly calendar.

- Treat yourself to new exercise clothes, if possible. If your old workout clothes make you feel heavy or look shabby, don't wear them. They won't make you want to exercise harder; they'll just make you feel bad about your body. Instead, buy some brand-new outfits in colors you like that make it easy to move, so you'll feel great about how you look.

- Dress to be ready to exercise. Want to excuse-proof your workout plans for the day? Here's one of my favorites boosters: When I get up in the morning, I don my exercise clothes (provided I have no business appointments) and wear them all day long. That way, I'm ready for my workout. Wearing my exercise clothes keeps me thinking and feeling "exercise." I'm less likely to talk myself out of it if I'm already suited up.

- Do your Naked Fitness workout with a friend. I've mentioned this already, but it is important enough to repeat. Knowing someone else is waiting will make you less likely to put off exercise or cancel it.

- Do it early. Studies have shown that we're more likely to skip a workout if we save it till after work or dinner, when we feel our most worn-out. Get up an hour or half-hour earlier than you normally would and do your routine. By working out early in the morning, you get your exercise session over with—and that feels good. Plus, exercise will energize you mentally and physically for the rest of the day.

- Mentally warm up. Take a lesson from competitive athletes. Start thinking about the benefits of your upcoming workout: the calories you'll burn, the muscles you'll firm, the stress-relieving chemicals that will flood your system, the way you'll look in your bikini in the summer. Imagine how invigorated you'll feel afterward. Replay this information in your head. Now go for it. You'll be amazed at what you can accomplish.

- Forgive yourself. If you have a week when you just don't have the energy, don't berate yourself for skipping your workout. Just don't let that week slide into two or three. Research shows that our reaction to a setback is more important than the setback itself. Being too critical or too easy on ourselves makes it more difficult to stick to a goal. The best way to handle a one-day lapse is to get back into your routine as soon as you can.

Warming Up

Before performing stretches and strength moves, do two to three minutes of easy cardio to get your heart rate up. I suggest the activities listed below; do one or a few.

- March in place. Pump your arms and lift your feet fully off the ground as high as is comfortable. Contract your glutes and hold in your abs.

- Dance. Put on some upbeat tunes and boogie around the living room.

- Jump rope. Bend your knees slightly, keep your abdominal muscles engaged, and land lightly on the balls of your feet. Get a steady rhythm going that you can maintain.

- Bounce on a trampoline. Many discount department stores as well as sporting goods stores, carry reliable exercise trampolines. This inexpensive piece of equipment is a fun way to warm up.

The Naked Fitness Routines

Depending on the results of your fitness test, you'll focus on one area of the spine—cervical, thoracic, lumbar—or a combination of these. This translates into your upper back, mid back, lower back, or a combination of alignment routines.

There are 10 stretches and 10 strengthening exercises for each routine. Before starting this or any other exercise program, it is important to see your doctor for a physical. Now, let's start your routine. Each routine should take approximately 15 minutes to complete. Perform the routine at least five days a week. Optimally, daily performance will yield faster results in improved posture and range of movement.

ROUTINE A:

UPPER BACK FOCUS—STRETCHES

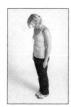 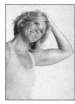 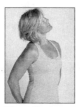

Chin Chest   Side Neck   Tilted Neck   Tilted Neck Stretch
Stretch   Stretch   Stretch Up   Down

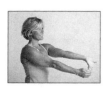   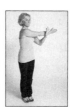

Single-Hand   Chin Rotation   Chest Stretch   Crossed Arm
Wrist/Wall Stretch   Low   Stretch

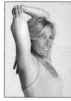 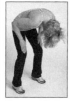

Overhead   Forward Roll
Triceps Stretch   Down

Chin Chest Stretch – Repeat 2 to 3 times.

Side Neck Stretch – Repeat 2 to 3 times on each side.

Tilted Neck Stretch Up – Repeat 2 to 3 times on each side.

Tilted Neck Stretch Down – Repeat 2 to 3 times on each side.

Single-Hand Wrist/Wall Stretch – Repeat 2 to 3 times on each side.

Chin Rotation – Repeat 2 times on each side.

Chest Stretch Low – Repeat 2 to 3 times.

Crossed Arm Stretch – Repeat 2 times on each side.

Overhead Triceps Stretch – Repeat 2 times on each side.

Forward Roll Down – Repeat 3 to 5 times.

ROUTINE A:

UPPER BACK FOCUS—STRENGTHENING MOVES

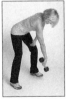

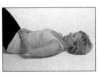

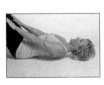
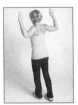

| Arm Circle Hangs | Chin Tilts | Wall Leans | Head Floor Leans | Shoulder Blade Squeeze |

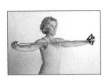

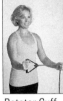
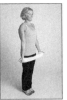

| Wide Pulls | Rotator Cuff Up | Rotator Cuff Side | Towel Twist Outs |

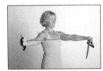

| Single-Arm Wide Pull, Thumbs Up | Single-Arm Wide Pull, Palms Down |

Arm Circle Hangs – Perform 8 repetitions clockwise and then counter clockwise.

Chin Tilts – Perform 8 to 12 repetitions.

Wall Leans – Perform 8 to 12 repetitions.

Head Floor Leans – Perform 8 to 12 repetitions.

Shoulder Blade Squeeze – Perform 3 to 5 repetitions.

Wide Pulls – Perform 8 to 12 repetitions.

Rotator Cuff Up – Perform 8 to 12 repetitions on each side.

Rotator Cuff Side – Perform 8 to 12 repetitions on each side.

Towel Twist Outs – Perform 8 to 12 repetitions.

Single-Arm Wide Pull, Thumbs Up – Perform 8 to 12 repetitions on each arm.

Single-Arm Wide Pull, Palms Down – Perform 8 to 12 repetitions on each arm.

ROUTINE B:

MID-BACK FOCUS—STRETCHES

 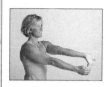 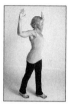

Side Neck   Single-Hand   Chest Stretch   Chest Stretch
Stretch   Wrist/Wall Stretch Low   High

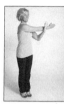   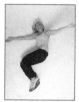

Crossed Arm   Arm Across   Figure 8 Arm   Bent Knee Side
Stretch   Low Stretch   Stretch   Stretch

 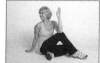

Cat to Cow   Spine Twist Up

Side Neck Stretch – Repeat 2 to 3 times on each side.

Single-Hand Wrist/Wall Stretch – Repeat 2 to 3 times on each side.

Chest Stretch Low – Repeat 2 to 3 times.

Chest Stretch High – Repeat 2 to 3 times.

Crossed Arm Stretch – Repeat 3 times on each side.

Arm Across Low Stretch – Repeat once on each side.

Figure 8 Arm Stretch – Perform four times on each side.

Bent Knee Side Stretch - Perform 2 to 3 times on each side.

Cat to Cow – Repeat 4 times.

Spine Twist Up – Repeat 4 times on each side.

ROUTINE B:

MID-BACK FOCUS—STRENGTHENING MOVES

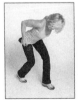

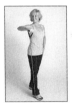

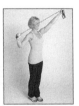

Shoulder Blade Squeeze, Row

Wide Pulls

Rotator Cuff Up

Rotator Cuff Side

Single-Arm Lat Pull Down

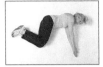
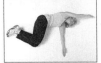

Shoulder Arm Circles

Side Plank on Knee

Knees Bent, Arms Reach Across

Rainbow Reaches

Superman

Shoulder Blade Squeeze with Row – Perform 3 to 5 repetitions.

Wide Pulls – Perform 8 to 12 repetitions.

Rotator Cuff Up – Perform 8 to 12 repetitions on each side.

Rotator Cuff Side – Perform 8 to 12 repetitions on each side.

Single-Arm Lat Pull Down – Perform 15 repetitions on each side.

Shoulder Arm Circles – Perform 10 circles in each direction.

Side Plank on Knee – Perform 8 to 12 repetitions.

Knees Bent, Arms Reach Across – Perform 5 to 8 repetitions on each side.

Rainbow Reaches – Perform 5 to 8 repetitions.

Superman – Perform 8 to 12 repetitions.

ROUTINE C:
LOWER BACK FOCUS—STRETCHES

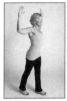 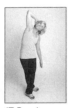 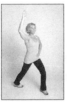 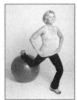 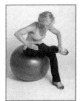

Chest Stretch   IT Band   Standing Hip   Hip Flexor   Seated Foot
High   Stretch   Flexor Stretch   Stretch Balance   Cross

 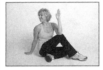 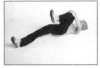 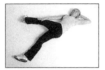

Double Knee to Side   Spine Twist Up   Knee to Chest Hip   Cross-Over Stretch
Stretch   Flexor Stretch

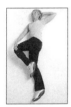

Sexy Spine

Chest Stretch High – Repeat 2 to 3 times.

IT Band Stretch – Perform 2 times on each side.

Standing Hip Flexor Stretch – Repeat 2 times on each side.

Hip Flexor Stretch Balance – Perform 2 to 3 times on each side.

Seated Foot Cross – Perform 3 times on each side.

Double Knee to Side Stretch – Repeat 2 times on each side.

Spine Twist Up -– Repeat 4 times on each side.

Knee to Chest Hip Flexor Stretch – Perform 2 to 3 times on each side.

Cross-Over Stretch – Perform once on each side.

Sexy Spine – Perform once on each side.

ROUTINE C:

LOWER BACK FOCUS—STRENGTHENING MOVES

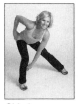 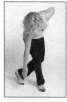 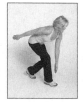 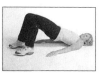

Side Lunge   Curtsy   Corner Mini   Bridge
                            Lunge

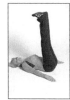 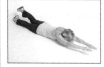 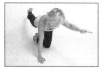

Bridge with Leg   Pelvic Tilt   Hamstring Curl
Lifts

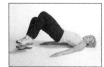 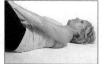

Toe Pulls   Swimmer   Pointer

Side Lunge – Alternate lunging from side to side for 20 repetitions.

Curtsy – Alternate from side to side for 20 repetitions.

Corner Mini Lunge – Perform 20 repetitions on the right and then 20 repetitions on the left.

Bridge – Perform 15 to 20 repetitions.

Bridge with Leg Lifts – Perform 20 alternating lifts.

Pelvic Tilt – Perform 10 to 15 repetitions.

Hamstring Curl – Perform 8 to 12 repetitions.

Toe Pulls, 3 positions – Perform 15 repetitions in each position.

Swimmer – Perform 20 repetitions.

Pointer – Perform 10 repetitions.

ROUTINE D:

TOTAL POSTURE—STRETCHES

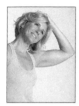 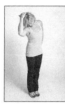 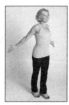 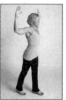 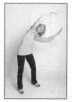

Side Neck   Hand Behind   Chest Stretch   Chest Stretch   Full Side
Stretch   Back Neck   Low   High   Bend Circle
                 Stretch

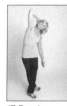 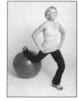 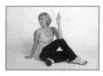 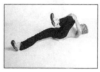

IT Band   Hip Flexor   Spine Twist Up   Knee to Chest Hip
Stretch   Stretch Balance   Flexor Stretch

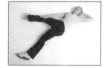

Cross-Over Stretch   Knee Tuck

Side Neck Stretch – Repeat 2 to 3 times on each side.

Hand Behind Back Neck Stretch – Repeat 2 times on each side.

Chest Stretch Low – Repeat 2 to 3 times.

Chest Stretch High – Repeat 2 to 3 times.

Full Side Bend Circle – Live-ilates™ stretch – Repeat 10 alternating circles.

IT Band Stretch – Repeat 2 times on each side.

Hip Flexor Stretch Balance– Repeat 2 times on each side.

Spine Twist Up – Repeat 4 times on each side.

Knee to Chest Hip Flexor Stretch – Perform 2 to 3 times on each side.

Cross-Over Stretch – Repeat once on each side.

Knee Tuck – Repeat 2 to 3 times on each side.

ROUTINE D:
TOTAL POSTURE—STRENGTHENING MOVES

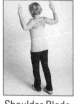
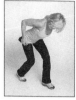
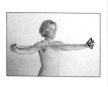

Shoulder Blade
Squeeze

Shoulder Blade
Squeeze, Row

Wide Pulls

Side Lunge

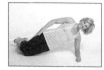
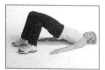

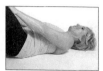

Side Plank on Knee

Bridge

Bridge with
Leg Lifts

Pelvic Tilt

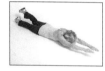
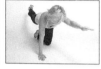

Swimmer

Pointer

Superman

Shoulder Blade Squeeze – Perform 3 to 5 repetitions.

Shoulder Blade Squeeze with Row – Perform 3 to 5 repetitions.

Wide Pulls – Perform 8 to 12 repetitions.

Side Lunge – Alternate lunging from side to side for 20 repetitions.

Side Plank on Knees – Perform 8 to 12 repetitions.

Bridge – Perform 15 to 20 repetitions.

Bridge with Leg Lifts – Perform 20 alternating lifts.

Pelvic Tilt – Perform 6 to 8 repetitions.

Pointer – Perform 20 repetitions.

Swimmer – Perform 20 repetitions.

Superman – Perform 8 to12 repetitions.

There you have it: simple, short, gentle-but-intense routines that will challenge your body, realign it, and get you into great shape.

6

WALK YOUR WAY
TO NAKED FITNESS

One of the secrets to success on Naked Fitness is walking two hours a day. You may be thinking to yourself, "Two hours a day? That's not possible!"

Before you protest, let me reassure you that walking two hours a day is not only doable, but honestly, is very easy to do. Nor is it time-consuming, because most of the time, you'll be "sneaking" your walk into your day. One of my clients, Brian N., is a great example.

Looking at Brian today, you'd never know the misery he's been through. After the scale maxed out 19 months ago, he began Naked Fitness. He was able to walk two hours a day by pacing around in his office while on conference calls. "In general, I walk around almost nonstop from 7:30 a.m. to 9 p.m. at night. On the weekends, I do an additional 60 minutes on an elliptical treadmill." Brian has lost a total of 75 pounds since starting his walking program, and no one can imagine how wonderful he feels.

Brian was able to sneak in two hours of walking by doing a lot of it as "incidental exercise." Incidental exercise is movement in the ordinary course of your day; for example, walking to the corner store, carrying groceries, or climbing stairs. If you live in a city, you'll probably get much more incidental exercise than do suburbanites, since the suburbs may lack sidewalks or put barriers in pedestrians' paths. The more people walk, the less overweight they are, and "high-walkability" neighborhoods have a lower incidence of obesity, according to studies.

There are many ways for you to reach the two-hour target. Some are familiar, but as more and more of my clients have started walking two hours a day, they've gotten very inventive about ways to do it. They suggest:

- Take the furthest parking space.

- Take the stairs.

- Walk your dog.

- Break up your walking into different activities: 30 minutes on a treadmill, 30 minutes on a stair-stepping machine, 30 minutes on an elliptical, or 30 minutes of walking during your lunch hour.

- Take your clients for a long walk instead of "doing lunch."

- Walk in place or on a treadmill while watching TV.

- Do as much of your daily business on foot, whether that is going to the post office or to the market.

- Walk around when you're waiting for a bus, airplane, train, or other appointment.

- Schedule walking meetings instead of group sit-downs in stuffy rooms.

- Walk while you shop; mall walking is a great way to sneak in exercise.

- Take some fun aerobics classes, such as Latin dancing or hip-hop. These count toward your daily walking quota because they are aerobic and help you burn fat.

- Walk while on your cellular or portable phone.

- Deliver memos on foot instead of emailing nearby coworkers.

- Compete in charity walks. The moment you enroll, you'll have a new sense of purpose and a concrete goal that will push you to achieve more.

Benefits

Walking is the easiest form of exercise and has the least amount of impact on the body, with the exception of swimming, which has big limitations (you need a pool, bathing suit, good weather [or an indoor pool], and so forth). Walking is easier on the lower extremities than jogging and is less strenuous than other aerobic exercises. It is ideal for sedentary people who are starting a fitness routine for the first time.

Walking is also a world-class deflabber: Mile for mile, you can burn as many calories walking as you would jogging, but with far less stress on your joints. And research shows that people who succeed at losing weight and keeping it off have one thing in common: They walk.

Here's a closer look at the benefits.

WEIGHT LOSS

If you commit to walking to tone up, slim down, and beautify your body, you won't be disappointed. As an aerobic exercise, walking effectively promotes weight loss because it burns calories. A casual or slow walker moves at a speed of about two miles per hour and burns about 200 calories per hour. Brisk walking or striding burns between 350 to 500 calories per hour at a rate of three-and-a-half to five miles per hour.

Walking has also been shown to raise metabolic rates for one to four hours after an exercise session. This means more energy is expended and more calories are burned. Also, studies have found that walking tends to curb the appetite.

SPOT-REDUCE YOUR WAISTLINE

It's true: You can spot-reduce your abs with walking! Researchers at the Washington University School of Medicine in St. Louis, Missouri, put a group of men and women, aged 60 to 70 on a 9- to 12-month exercise program that consisted of walking or jogging. On average, the subjects exercised 45 minutes several times a week. By the end of the study, both the men and the women had lost weight. But get this: Most of their weight was shed from the abdominal area. This all goes to show that a simple exercise program like walking can melt off abdominal fat, which creeps on as we get older. Based on this information, the best flab-busting aerobics for your midsection include walking, jogging or running, and treadmill exercise.

IMPROVE HEART HEALTH

For years, people thought that only sweaty, heart-pounding exercise was aerobic enough to do your heart any good. But that concept began to collapse when scientists discovered that people who walked briskly for 30 minutes or more a day had a noticeably reduced incidence of heart disease.

One of the major factors was a dramatic Boston study analyzing more than 120,000 women, which appeared in the *New England Journal of Medicine* in 1999. It showed that walking three or more hours a week cut women's threat of heart disease by a striking 30 percent; five or more hours cut it by an even more impressive 40 percent.

During walking, or any aerobic exercise, your oxygen consumption increases. Subsequently, circulatory and respiratory function are improved. People who have suffered heart attacks are advised to walk as part of their cardiac rehabilitation to strengthen and condition the heart. Many studies are now linking the benefits of walking and other aerobic exercises to a reduction in high blood pressure, lower blood cholesterol, and better control of diabetes. A 12-year Harvard University study found that brisk walking increases longevity. Just think, we can move our beautiful, naked bodies through space and receive the most amazing benefit of all: extended life!

TONE YOUR BONES AND JOINTS

As our bodies age, our bones tend to become more porous due to a loss of bone mass and tissue, resulting in a loss of bone strength. Weakened bones are brittle and more prone to fractures—a disease known as osteoporosis. The progression of osteoporosis can be prevented or slowed down by walking because the exercise, along with an appropriate calcium intake, ramps up the amount of minerals in the bones.

Walking also eases osteoarthritis, the most common form of arthritis. An Australian study published in *Arthritis Research & Therapy* in 2010 found that "progressive walking" combined with a glucosamine supplement improved the symptoms of osteoarthritis. The researchers observed 36 arthritis patients age 42 to 73. All patients received the supplement for 6 weeks and continued to take it during the 12-week walking program. Of the 36 participants, 17 walked five days a week; 19 walked three days a week (two reps of 1,500 steps). Both groups had significant improvement in their osteoarthritis symptoms.

SLEEP MORE SOUNDLY

Poor sleep is a serious problem. Even one night of insufficient or restless sleep can result in irritability and an inability to concentrate. Various studies indicate that establishing a chronic sleep debt can depress your immune system. That means you're more likely to catch viruses. And a lack of sleep can also be downright dangerous. The Department of Transportation estimates that up to 100,000 motor vehicle accidents a year occur because drivers become drowsy or fall asleep at the wheel.

Yet, like any problem, sleep disorders can be managed and conquered. One of the best ways is through walking. At the Stanford University School of Medicine, researchers studied 29 women and 14 men, age 50 to 76 who were sedentary and free of cardiovascular disease and who said they had trouble sleeping. The group underwent 30 to 40 minutes of low-impact aerobics or brisk walking four times a week for 16 weeks. Those who exercised slept almost an hour longer each night and fell asleep in half the time it took before they participated in the study. However, don't work out less than three hours before going to bed, as it may stimulate the body rather than calm it down.

STRESS LESS

Stress, which manifests itself as wear and tear on the body, must be released to avoid permanent illness or disease. Walking offers a good physical outlet, which is necessary to release the chemical build-up caused by a bad day at the office or other tense situations. Plus, it stimulates the brain to produce mood-boosting chemicals called endorphins. You will feel good about yourself and therefore be more able to face the demands and pressures of life.

IMPROVED ATTITUDE AND MENTAL FUNCTIONING

Anxiety and tension are best released through exercise. Walkers usually experience mood elevations and a sense of well-being after a brisk work-out. Consistent walking programs also have helped reduce and eliminate depression.

Posture and Alignment Tips While Walking

As you get started on your walking program, focus on the following five points of posture. They will help reinforce your posture and improve your alignment. The old song, "Head, shoulders, knees and toes, knees and toes" should be your mantra while walking—and throw in belly since it's there!

1. **Head Position.** Keep your eyes looking forward but slightly down. Keep your chin parallel to the ground and the base of your head over your tailbone.

2. **Chest.** Keep your arms swinging along your sides and your chest open, with your collar bones and sternum lifted slightly.

3. **Abdominals.** Walk tall while drawing your belly button into your spine. All this requires is a slight engagement (flexing) of your core (the center of your body). This position keeps your pelvis from tipping forward and helps you avoid lower back strain.

4. **Knees.** While walking, many people rest through the knee joint, making the knee bow slightly backward in a curved position. Instead, keep tension in your thighs by slightly drawing your kneecap upward when you walk. If this is difficult at first, practice it while standing.

5. **Toes.** Make sure your toes point forward in your walking alignment. Even if your feet seem to naturally turn outward, you have the power to keep your toes pointed forward. Your muscles have probably been trained to angle outward due to tight hip flexors from sitting long periods or overuse of forward motion cardio like walking or running. When your heel lands in front, make sure the toes are pointing forward. Think of your toe positions like a car with alignment issues: It will run, but unless corrected, eventually it will give you some problems.

Also, swing your arms naturally by your sides or, to increase the intensity, bend your elbows to 90 degrees and drive them forward. Keep your hands empty and unclenched (clip your MP3 player or water bottle to a fitness belt).

Getting the Most from Your Walk

In addition to using the five points of posture to get the most from your walk, here are some other things you can do to mix it up, get more calorie burn, and improve your alignment.

WALK AND RUN IN INTERVALS

An interval is a brief bout of intense physical activity such as a sprint alternated with a longer period of rest or lighter exercise like walking. You might alternate two minutes of slower-paced walking with one minute of fast walking or jogging. With this type of interval training, you can change the way the interval affects your body. It revs up fat-burning in cells, burns more calories, boosts your good cholesterol, and enhances your cardiovascular fitness.

This form of interval training is a great way to build up to jogging or running. Gradually decrease your walking intervals and increase your jogging intervals, and you'll be doing a full run before you know it.

GO FOR THE GRADE

Use incline, grade, or hills to challenge yourself. Upping the incline to a 10 percent grade can have significant effects on your energy consumption. My client Kristin found that when she walked at 2.8 mph on a flat grade, her heart rate was about 120 beats per minute. When she upped the incline to a 10 percent grade at that same pace, her heart rate shot up to 156, which was the upper end of her training zone. This increase represents a significant change in calorie burn—about 25 to 30 percent per hour. If she couldn't maintain that grade, she would reduce the intensity by lowering the grade and try for 2:1-minute intervals.

An additional tip: To avoid straining your leg muscles when you're tackling a steep hill, lean forward and bend your knees slightly.

TRY WALK-ILATES™

Once you've done a considerable amount of daily walking, you'll find that the following variations will help you improve your walk, strengthen and stretch the muscles around the hips, and improve total movement patterns.

HEEL WALKING

Walk on your heels for 30 paces at least three times during your walk. Heel walking provides a natural stretch on your calf muscles and helps strengthen the shin muscles. The balanced muscle patterns can help prevent plantar fasciitis, a common ailment in walkers.

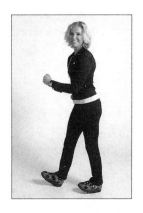

SIDE WALKING

Walk sideways for at least 30 seconds, leading with the outer thigh and closing the step with the opposite leg. Then, return to your forward movement. Repeat this drill every minute for at least six minutes to help strengthen and stretch your IT band, inner and outer thighs, and gluteal and hip rotator muscle groups. Be sure to alternate the starting foot.

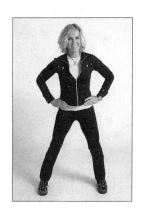

TRY WALK-ILATES™ (continued)

CROSS-OVER WALKING

Walk sideways with the back leg crossing over and then behind the lead leg. Some people call this move a "grapevine." The pattern can help strengthen the smaller muscles supporting and stabilizing the hip and knee joints.

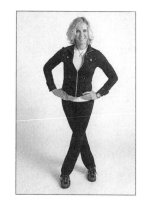

WAIST-WHITTLER WALKING

Walking with arms bent and elbows out to the side at shoulder height, increase your upper body rotation and walk a little bit slower. Perform this movement pattern for one to two minutes each time you step out.

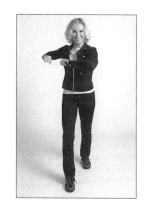

TOE-TURNED HEEL ROCK

Starting in a split stance (one foot behind the other) with the back foot turned inward, roll the heel up and down keeping the back leg straight and the front knee bent. This heel lift and stretch will help strengthen the calf muscles and stretch the hip flexors. Perform 10 repetitions on each side.

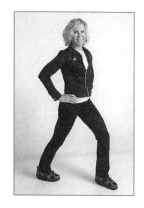

CHANGE THE TERRAIN

You can walk on just about any surface. However, for extra benefits, try to vary the surfaces you walk on. Trails provide a softer surface and a pleasant environment so workouts stay interesting. Walking on sand is the most strenuous but burns the most calories. Street surfaces allow you to walk faster, but lights, curbs, and traffic make it difficult to walk unimpeded for long periods.

Some advice about safety: There are many safety precautions to heed as a walker, especially in the city. Know the rules of the road, wear bright clothing, don't walk in unfamiliar, desolate places, and let people know where you are.

WEAR CORE-BALANCING SHOES

Try a core-balancing shoe—the type advertised to tone up your legs and lower body. These shoes provide an unstable walking platform and specially designed mid-soles. The point is to increase muscle contractions and mimic the effects of walking on soft sand. As you walk, your heel sinks into the soft foam insole before rolling forward onto the forefoot and pushing off with the toes. This way of walking activates more muscles in the legs, buttocks, and back while employing the core muscles to stabilize your steps. The result is a better walking workout, for more efficient toning and strength.

Whether you wear core-balancing shoes or other fitness shoes, walking requires a correct-fitting, comfortable pair of shoes. Any low-heeled shoe that offers adequate cushioning, reinforcement in the back around the heel area, and flexibility in the toe area will do the trick. Also, be sure to replace them every 300 to 500 miles. Even if your footwear looks fine, its shock-absorbing material will probably be depleted—a state of disrepair that could make you prone to injury.

WALK WITH POLES

A conditioning activity known as "fitness pole walking," or "Nordic walking," can help you lose weight and build cardiovascular conditioning. Pole walking uses cross-country ski poles that have been converted for walking. This technique shifts weight away from your lower limbs and makes walking safer.

A plus is that you use so much more muscle mass that your metabolic rate is quite a bit higher, so you get a shorter, much more intensive workout. Instead of working just your leg muscles, pole walking also exercises all the main muscles in the upper body, including your abdominals, biceps, forearms, pectorals, and spinal rectors. Additionally, it creates far less impact with the ground than running.

As you push down gently on the poles, you create more resistance as you walk and build upper body and core strength as well. Yet the poles themselves also take weight off your joints, making it ideal for overweight people with joint problems beginning a walking regimen. Add up- and downhill grades to the course, and you've got yourself a pretty good workout.

Dozens of studies have been conducted on the benefits of pole walking: It increases upper-body endurance, burns more calories than regular walking, and is an effective rehab tool for patients with limited shoulder mobility. Walking poles are available at many sporting goods stores.

TRY TREADMILLS

Treadmills provide a great way for you to walk, jog, or run indoors at home or in a gym. You can adjust the speed of the treadmill according to your level of fitness and increase the speed gradually as you become more conditioned. You can also adjust the grade, or slope, of the treadmill to make the exercise harder, like you're jogging or running uphill. Some computerized treadmills let you choose programs in which the speed and grade automatically change while you're on the machine. On a treadmill you can do high-intensity speed intervals too.

To burn more calories, try swinging your arms while you walk on the treadmill. Research shows that vigorous arm swinging increases your calorie-burning potential by 50 percent, and it gives your upper body a good workout.

USE STAIRCLIMBING MACHINES

Like many mechanized aerobic machines, stairclimbers provide instant feedback about calories burned, heart rate, and other variables. You can set the level of difficulty too. These machines work the large muscles of the lower body, adding to the intensity of the effort, and increase leg strength.

WALK IN WATER

Walking in water has several advantages over dry-land workouts. The weightless effect you experience in water gives your body greater flexibility than it has on land. According to experts, because your weight in water is a tenth of what it would be on land, your range of motion is much greater.

Another bonus of water is that it gives you 12 times more resistance when you move than air does. That resistance gives your muscles a workout similar to what occurs when you train with weights, but without the added stress to muscles and joints. There also is a low incidence of high-impact injuries when you work out in water. In addition, a recent study showed that water walkers moving 1.5 to 2 mph got the same health benefits that land walkers did at a 3.5 to 8 mph pace.

BREAK IT UP

An easy way to fit in your walking is to walk 10 minutes before and after each meal (that's a total of 60 minutes). Then walk again 30 minutes prior to going to bed and 30 minutes upon arising. This game plan will help you get in your two hours of walking daily.

What's a Good Pace?

Pace depends on your level of conditioning, walking experience, and goals. Here are some guidelines to help you.

- For overall good health, walk comfortably at a steady pace, breathing easily. You should feel like you've exercised without feeling exhausted.

- To lose weight, try the interval method I described above. Your breathing should be manageable yet somewhat challenged at the moderate pace and harder on the intervals.

- To relieve stress, maintain a comfortable, rhythmic pace that allows you to focus on one of your mantras or your breathing.

Measuring Your Time and Miles

You'll want to eventually walk two hours daily, so it's a good idea to keep track of your walking time. You can record your time in your journal or in the daily walking log in Appendix E, or measure your progress with a pedometer, a pager-sized device that senses your body's movement and measures how many steps you take.

Walking two hours a day is roughly equal to 15,000 steps a day and will burn nearly 750 calories daily. That amount of walking could lead to a 7-pound weight loss within a month without any other changes.

The goal of Naked Fitness is to work your way up to two hours, or 15,000 steps, a day. While that may sound like a lot, it turns out that even die-hard couch potatoes log about 2,000 to 4,000 steps a day— about one to two miles—just doing their minimum basic daily activities. A typical busy woman may do 5,000 to 6,000 steps a day.

Pedometers are available in drugstores, sporting goods stores, and online, and range in price from $5 to $75 and up. Honestly, the more expensive they are, the more accurately they count your steps.

Many are programmed using your height, weight, age, and the length of your stride. Once you've input that information, the device will not only count your steps but tell you the distance you have walked, how many calories you have burned, and how long you have been walking.

You can wear some pedometers clipped to your waistband, while you can carry others in your pocket or a bag.

Using a Heart-Rate Monitor

Another gadget worth investing in is a heart-rate monitor. A monitor costs less than $100 and come with instructions.

This device helps gauge your intensity and your progress. Your heart rate is a window to your cardiovascular fitness. Let's say you can walk 1 mile in 15 minutes at a heart rate of 135 beats per minute. Six weeks from now, you may be able to cover more ground—say 1.1 miles—

in the same amount of time at the same heart rate. This means you've become more fit because you can accomplish more work without putting additional stress on your body.

The manual method of gauging your heart rate involves math. Subtract your age from 220. This is your maximum heart rate per minute. Multiply this number by 0.50 to figure the low end and by 0.85 to determine the high end of your target heart rate. You should stay within these limits. If you exceed your ideal heart rate with very high-intensity exercise, like sprinting, the workout becomes anaerobic, meaning it requires more energy than your body can supply. Your body then starts burning glycogen, which is muscles' food. It also produces lactic acid, which makes you feel sore after a workout. So you want to stay in your target range because this is the level at which the most fat is burned.

Starting Your Walk

You should incorporate two important activities into every walking program: a warm-up and a cool-down period. Many people confuse warming up with stretching out muscles, but they are not the same thing. Your walk should begin at a slow, casual pace for the first five minutes or so; this is considered a warm-up. Once you're in the groove, increase your pace. During the last five minutes of your walk, slow your pace and stride to allow yourself to cool down naturally. Then treat yourself to a tall glass of water.

Work Your Way Up

If you're just starting a walking program, begin the first week by walking 20 minutes three times a week. For the next few weeks, increase your time to 30 minutes. As you feel more energetic and fit, add an extra session or two to your weekly walking program. Try to add more walking minutes and/or steps each day. Vary the duration, intensity, and terrain, plus try different walking techniques to keep your body challenged.

A body that looks wonderful naked, better physical and mental health, more energy, and weight and stress reduction all are gifts from your feet to you. Most important, walking is fun. If you aren't already walking for fitness, doesn't it make sense to start today?

PART 3

Naked Nutrition

7

THE NAKED FITNESS
NUTRITION PRINCIPLES

The most effective way to knock off the pounds and keep them off is with a plan that emphasizes a variety of foods, controls calories, and includes regular exercise. The Naked Fitness Nutrition Plan, along with your specially designed workout, is that approach. Based on scientific evidence about weight loss, it's healthy and energizing, plus simple and easy to follow. Stick with it, and before long, you'll experience a level of fitness that you can see and feel—in your clothes and out of them.

When you start a diet, you want to see results right away in how you look and how you feel. That's because our society is geared toward the immediate; we want things and we want them now. The same is true for weight loss. We get impatient when the pounds don't come off fast enough, so it seems so much easier to give up than to go on.

This plan is designed to produce quick results, not because it starves you down to size, but because its carefully designed balance of food and exercise adjusts your body metabolically so that you burn fat, day in and day out.

Here's a detailed look at how and why the Naked Fitness Nutrition Plan works.

A Healthy Nutritional Balance

Weight-loss diets frequently get criticized because they supposedly do not furnish a healthy supply of nutrients, and this is certainly true of many diets. But in far too many cases—and research bears this out—everyday eating habits tend to be more unbalanced, with an insufficient supply of critical nutrients, than most diets are. Plus, the average person simply doesn't eat nutritiously enough to meet even the basic daily requirements of vitamins, minerals, and fiber according to several studies. Consider, for example, a typical American diet:

Breakfast: One super-large bagel, one cup of orange juice, and one cup of coffee with a tablespoon of half-and-half

Lunch: Ham and cheese sandwich, small bag of potato chips, one medium apple, and a can of cola

Mid-Afternoon Snack: Cookies and a can of cola

Fast-Food Dinner: Supersized cheeseburger and French fries

Evening Snack: A bowl of vanilla ice cream

Although it supplies plenty of energy (2,264 calories), this menu is deficient in several vital nutrients: calcium, a bone-building mineral; magnesium, important to heart health; selenium, widely recognized as a cancer preventive; vitamin A, vital for disease-fighting; and vitamin E, a nutrient that confers a wide range of health-protective benefits. This menu is critically low in fiber too (barely 10 grams), supplying less than half of what we normally need each day. Plus, more than 40 percent of its calories come from fat. Fat intake should be no more than 30 percent of your daily calories.

Often, a person will go on a weight-loss diet, forsaking junk food, and in doing so, start eating more nutritiously than ever before. So diets should not take all of the blame for Americans' poor nutritional habits.

I have devised the Naked Fitness Nutrition Plan to provide a healthy combination of basic nutrients—protein, carbohydrates, fats, vitamins, and minerals—that your body requires to burn fat efficiently.

Foods in Fat-Burning Proportions

The Naked Fitness Nutrition Plan emphasizes proportions of foods that studies have shown to help peel off pounds and banish them for good. Proportionately, this plan is high in protein (25 to 30 percent of total daily calories), low to moderate in carbohydrates (40 to 50 percent of total calories), and moderate in fat (around 30 percent of total calories). This approach suits the needs of active people, stimulates fat metabolism, and supplies the nutrients required to support your health while losing weight.

A High-Protein Plan for Burning Calories

Protein is to your body what a wood frame is to your house or steel is to a bridge. Nutritionally, it is the basic, most important building material in your body, essential to high-level health because of its role in growth and maintenance. Your body breaks down protein from food into nutrient fragments called amino acids and reshuffles them into new protein to build and rebuild tissue, including body-firming muscle. Protein also keeps your immune system functioning up to par, helps carry nutrients throughout the body, has a hand in forming hormones, and is involved in important enzyme reactions such as digestion. I've designed the Naked Fitness Nutrition Plan to be high in protein because protein stimulates the reduction of body fat.

Proteins on this plan include fish, meats, poultry, eggs, and certain calcium-rich dairy products.

You'll eat protein in ample amounts—around 30 percent of your total daily calories. When provided in your diet at generally higher levels, protein can be nicknamed a "fat burner" for two important reasons.

First, your body requires ample protein to develop and maintain body-firming muscle. If you don't get enough protein, your body can start breaking down muscle tissue for the provision of energy. Consequently, you'll lose metabolically active muscle, and this will sabotage your fat-loss efforts.

Second, protein boosts your metabolism by stepping up the action of your thyroid gland. (One of the main functions of the thyroid is to regulate metabolism.) This benefit of a high-protein diet was observed in a study of dieters conducted by the University of Illinois at Urbana-Champaign, released in 2001.

In this study, 24 middle-aged women went on a 1,700-calorie-a-day diet for 10 weeks. Half followed a higher-carbohydrate, lower-protein diet—55 percent carbohydrates, 15 percent protein, and 30 percent fat. The other half followed a high-protein diet of 40 percent carbohydrates, 30 percent protein, and 30 percent fat.

Both groups lost the same amount of weight (16 pounds on the average), but the composition of that weight differed greatly. The high-protein group shed 12.3 pounds of pure pudge and only 1.7 pounds of lean muscle, while the other dieters lost 10.4 pounds of fat and 3 pounds of muscle. Translation: High protein means better, more figure-flattering fat loss. With a higher-protein diet, you don't have to sacrifice body-firming muscle. Also important in this study, the researchers detected an increase in the thyroid function of the high-protein dieters, and this was concrete evidence of protein's metabolism-boosting effect.

Protein has such a powerful effect on weight loss that if you replace some of the carbohydrate in your diet with protein, your body will become a fat-burning machine. This was clearly demonstrated in a study conducted at the Research Department of Human Nutrition in Copen-hagen, Denmark. Overweight and obese volunteers were placed on either a high-carbohydrate diet (protein comprised just 12 percent of the total daily calories) or a high-protein diet (25 percent of the daily calories were derived from protein). The study lasted six months. At its conclusion, the high-protein group had lost nearly 20 pounds, on the average while the high-carbohydrate group had lost only about half that amount—11 pounds on the average. But here is something equally amazing: Of the pounds lost in the high-protein group, 17 pounds were pure fat, compared to just 9 pounds in the high-carbohydrate group. Again, a high-protein diet trims away more fat than any other approach appears to do.

The upshot is that with more protein in your diet, in the right balance, you can almost double your weight-loss and fat-burning results!

Based on this important knowledge, the Naked Fitness Nutrition Plan will result in significant fat loss.

The Carbohydrate Question

Carbohydrates are one of the biggest variables in weight loss, because they supply a lot of calories. Carbohydrates are classified as either simple or complex. Simple sugars are found in candies, syrups, fruit juices, and processed foods, and complex carbohydrates are found in whole grains, beans, and vegetables. This classification is based on the molecular structure of the carbohydrate: simple carbohydrates are constructed of either single or double molecules of sugar, and complex carbohydrates are made of multiple numbers of sugar molecules.

Carbs, particularly simple carbs, trigger the release of insulin, a hormone that "tells" your body to convert calories to fat instead of burning them off. This means the body starts storing energy as fat; the end result of eating too many carbohydrates is obesity. A high intake of carbohydrates over time can also increase the risk of becoming diabetic due to the increased production of insulin from high glucose intake.

Keeping your carbohydrates in the moderate range will thus help you burn fat faster because you'll keep insulin levels in check. You will not avoid all carbohydrates on the Naked Fitness Nutrition Plan, because high-fiber vegetables such as lettuce and broccoli (yes, these vegetables do contain carbohydrates) have more fiber, vitamins, and nutrients than other carbs and are associated with lower rates of hypertension, cancer, arthritis, and diabetes. Low-fiber carbohydrates like bananas are high in potassium, and tomatoes are rich in vitamins and linked to the prevention of prostate cancer.

Fiber and Fat-Burning

Fiber is what your grandmother used to call "roughage." It is the food component that keeps us regular, and certain foods are packed with it.

The "push" response of your intestines depends on adequate fiber in your diet. Low amounts of fiber are linked to dozens of medical problems including heart disease, some cancers, diabetes, diverticulosis, and gall-stones. High amounts of fiber, on the other hand, as part of an overall healthy diet, help reduce blood cholesterol levels and may lower the risk of heart disease. Fiber-containing foods provide a feeling of fullness with fewer calories.

As for weight control, high-fiber eating helps peel off pounds and banish them for good. Fiber does this mainly by curtailing your food intake. Specifically, fibrous foods provide bulk and stimulate the release of appetite-suppressing hormones. As a result, you feel full while eating a meal, so you're less tempted to overeat.

High-fiber foods also take longer to chew, so your meals last longer. That's a plus, since it takes about 20 minutes after starting a meal for your body to send signals that it's full. And, when eaten with other nutrients, fiber slows the rate of digestion, curbing your appetite between meals. Fiber also increases the time it takes for food to move through your intestinal system, meaning fewer calories are left to be stored as fat.

On the Naked Fitness Nutrition Plan you'll eat 25 to 35 grams of fiber daily. It will come from fruits, vegetables, beans and legumes, and a few high-fiber starches, namely high-fiber tortillas and pearled barley.

Beneficial Fats

Fats are the black-hatted guys of nutrition, the most demonized of all nutrients. But do fats really deserve all that bad press?

Sure, a few fats do pose health risks, including the saturated fats found in tropical oils such as coconut oil and trans fats, which are synthetic fats found mostly in margarine, vegetable shortening, and processed foods. All of these fats have been associated with an increased risk of heart disease. In addition, saturated fat has been implicated in prostate cancer, and trans fats in breast cancer.

Fortunately, though, there are more good fats than bad ones. To understand the health importance of good fats, let's start with a quick nutrition lesson.

POLYUNSATURATED AND MONOUNSATURATED FATS

Good fats fall under a general classification of unsaturated fats. There are two types of unsaturated fats: polyunsaturated and monounsaturated. Oils such as safflower, sunflower, corn, soybean, and fish oils are polyunsaturated fats. They contain alpha linolenic acid and linoleic acid, referred to as "essential fatty acids," or EFAs for short. Required for normal body function, EFAs must be supplied by your diet since the body cannot make them on its own.

From alpha linolenic acid, found in walnuts and dark, leafy greens, your body synthesizes two other important fatty acids: eicosapentaenoic acid (EPA) and docosahexaenoic acid (DHA). These fatty acids, along with alpha linolenic acid, are referred to as omega-3 fatty acids, a term that describes their molecular structure. You can also obtain EPA and DHA directly from cold-water fish, flaxseed, and omega-3–enriched eggs (eggs from chickens fed fish meal or flax meal).

Linoleic acid is an omega-6 fatty acid involved in a number of important body processes. It is found mostly in vegetable oils, nuts, and seeds.

Monounsaturated fats are plentiful in shellfish and cold-water fish such as salmon, mackerel, halibut, black cod, and rainbow trout.

Your body converts the essential fatty acids available from good fats into "prostaglandins" in the body. Prostaglandins are hormone-like chemicals that regulate numerous processes, including blood pressure, normal blood clot formation, blood lipids, immunity, inflammation in response to injury, and many other vital functions. There are not-so-friendly prostaglandins in the body too, synthesized mostly from saturated fats. Fortunately, you can keep these prostaglandins at bay by cutting back on your intake of saturated fats.

THE ROLE OF FAT

Fat helps your body transport, absorb, and store vitamins A, D, E, and K, collectively known as the fat-soluble vitamins. You need vitamin A for a strong immune system, vitamin D to absorb calcium, vitamin E to protect cells, and vitamin K for normal blood clotting. Without adequate fat in your diet, you won't get the maximum benefits from these vitamins. Although fairly tasteless itself, fat imparts enticing flavor and aroma to foods, thus stimulating your appetite. You experience this every time you smell bacon frying or cookies baking.

Dietary fat is an essential nutrient that your body requires to help form the structures of cell membranes, regulate metabolism, and provide a source of energy for exercise and activity. Along with carbohydrates, fat is a vital fuel source for your body.

THE LOW-FAT FOOD MYTH

For decades, we were taught that to lose weight, we had to slash the amount of dietary fat in our diets. Since the 1980s, Americans have reduced their fat consumption, but at the same time, they got fatter. More than 60 percent of our population is now considered overweight or obese. Cutting the fat from our diets was clearly not the magic answer to weight loss.

Scientists studying this alarming trend probed the reasons. What could explain this confusing phenomenon? After much research, they discovered that people had been replacing the fat in their diets with too many carbohydrates. This was the cause of the expanding waistlines of the American public, along with the fact that Americans are becoming increasingly inactive. So from a nutritional standpoint, carbohydrates are among the prime culprits in weight gain, and dietary fat shoulders far less of the blame. Also, as noted above, eating too many carbs stimulates the formation of body fat.

What this means to you is that, unless you are under a physician-supervised low-fat diet to control a specific disease, you do not have to worry about slashing dietary fat to unrealistic levels while on the Naked Fitness Nutrition Plan. In fact, a growing catalog of studies suggests that you can lose weight on a diet in which 30 percent of your total calories come from fat. This quantity of fat is considered moderate.

In one fascinating study, conducted at Brigham and Women's Hospital and Harvard Medical School, researchers looked into the long-term weight-loss effects of following a moderate-fat diet compared to following a low-fat diet in a group of overweight men and women. After 18 months, those on the moderate-fat program lost ten pounds, while the low-fat dieters gained more than six pounds! Plus, the people on the moderate-fat program found it easier to comply with the diet.

There are two reasons why you will find it much easier to stick to a moderate-fat diet: flavor and appetite. As I said before, although fairly tasteless itself, fat imparts enticing flavor and aroma to foods. Food simply tastes better when it contains fat.

Fat also has an appetite-suppressing effect. That's because it is slow to digest and thus makes you feel full after you've eaten a meal. Fat also stimulates the intestinal wall to secrete an appetite-control hormone called cholecystokinin (CCK), which acts on nerves in your stomach and slows the rate of digestion. CCK is also released by the hypothalamus, the body's appetite control center. The net effect of CCK's release in the body is to tell your brain that you're full.

Taking all of this important information into account, the Naked Fitness Nutrition Plan supplies roughly 30 percent of your daily calories from fat. Most of the allowable fat on this diet comes from nuts and salad dressings of all types.

Walnuts: The Get-Slim Secret

One source of fat I emphasize on the Naked Fitness Nutrition Plan is the walnut. Walnuts are the only nuts that contain a significant amount of omega-3 fatty acids, which along with other essential fats, are necessary for good health. The beneficial fats found in walnuts help keep your blood sugar stable for a few hours after they are consumed, which in turn promotes weight loss. Basically, when your blood sugar level is balanced, your body can burn calories from its own fat stores, whereas when your blood sugar level is imbalanced, you crave carbohydrates and sugar.

Walnuts also contain potassium, which aids in muscle development. The more lean muscle you have, the better your body burns fat. It's also packed with protein and contains a moderate amount of calories and fat (an ounce—approximately 24 nuts—has 6 grams of protein, 160 calories, and 14 grams of fat).

So one of your best fat bets for weight loss is the walnut. What's more, walnuts help protect the heart, fight cancer, and reduce symptoms of inflammatory diseases like arthritis.

Other Nuts and Treats

You'll also be able to enjoy almonds and some types of trail mix on the Naked Fitness Nutrition Plan. The almond is a very well-balanced food. It contains the right kind of fats (monounsaturated and some poly-unsaturated fats) and thus may help lower low-density lipoprotein (LDL), or "bad" cholesterol, levels while not touching high-density lipoprotein, or "good" cholesterol, levels or contributing to weight gain.

One ounce of almonds (about 20 to 30 nuts) contains 35 percent of your daily required value of vitamin E, a powerful antioxidant. Anti-oxidants are thought to protect the body's cells from damaging oxygen free radicals, which promote heart disease, cancer, and aging. Also, two phytochemicals found in almonds—quercetin and kaempferol—have been shown to inhibit the growth of lung, prostate, and breast tumors in laboratory studies. With three grams of fiber per ounce, the almond has the highest amount of fiber of any seed or nut.

Trail mix makes a healthy snack. Compared to many packaged snacks, this option is lower in calories and satisfies you for a longer time. Try dried apricots and almonds, dried mangoes and Brazil nuts, and dried figs and walnuts. But be moderate. Eat no more than an ounce of trail mix a few times a week.

Vitamins for a Healthy Naked Body

Required by your body in tiny amounts, vitamins play important roles in the metabolism of carbohydrates, proteins, and fats. The vita-mins you need daily are found in the Naked Fitness Nutrition Plan as follows:

Vitamin A: Green leafy vegetables, carrots, fruits, and eggs
Vitamin B-complex: Protein foods, legumes, fruits, and vegetables

Vitamin C: Fruits and vegetables
Vitamin D: Calcium-rich dairy foods
Vitamin E: Green leafy vegetables, walnuts, nuts, and eggs

Minerals for Metabolism

Like vitamins, minerals play a role in metabolism. But a major difference between the two nutrients is that minerals are constituents of bodily structures such as bone, cartilage, and teeth and provide their hardness and strength. While vitamins help manufacture these structures, they do not become part of the structures themselves.

The minerals you need daily are found in the Naked Fitness Nutrition Plan as follows:

Iron: Meats, poultry, eggs, walnuts, green leafy vegetables, and fruits
Calcium: Greek-style yogurt, cottage cheese, salmon, green leafy vegetables, and broccoli
Copper: Meats, shellfish, and walnuts
Magnesium: Meats and walnuts
Phosphorus: Meats, poultry, fish, and walnuts
Potassium: Fruits and vegetables
Selenium: Fish and eggs
Zinc: Shellfish, meats, and vegetables

Multiple Meals = Faster Metabolism

While following the Naked Fitness Nutrition Plan, you'll eat multiple meals each day. This means at least four to five meals and snacks a day. So on this plan, you'll forgo your usual three squares a day and eat four or five times: three main meals plus one or two snacks.

Research shows that eating multiple meals (including snacks) increases "thermogenesis," the production of heat by the body as it digests and absorbs food. During thermogenesis, metabolism speeds up.

Increased meal frequency also stimulates fat burning, preserves body-firming muscle, and reduces your appetite.

What About Calories?

The Naked Fitness Nutrition Plan reduces your calorie intake to allow you to lose weight at an appreciable speed. All diets boil down to a simple formula: Eat fewer calories than you burn. Break that rule, and all the carb-cutting, fat-banning eating in the world won't make a bit of difference. This is why weight-loss experts are now advocating a back-to-basics approach: calorie counting.

Exactly what is a calorie anyway? It's a measure of energy in food. Technically, one calorie is the amount of energy it takes to raise the temperature of one gram of water by one degree Celsius. Calories are like gasoline. The same way that gas makes your car go, calories fuel your body.

After you eat a meal, your digestive system breaks down the chemical bonds that hold food molecules together. Energy contained in those bonds is released and available for use. Your body uses that energy to fuel everything from basic activities like breathing, thinking, and growing hair to bigger tasks like carrying a pregnancy or doing your exercise program.

However, when you don't use the calories you've taken in (maybe you decide to skip your workout one day), those calories get escorted to your liver to refill your glycogen stores. Glycogen is your body's easy-access energy reserve. Because your body stores it, you don't have to eat continuously to keep your body energized. Still, glycogen is depleted every three to four hours. When your liver is holding as much glycogen as it can, some of it is passed on to muscles for short-term storage (to be used as needed to move your body and get you through a workout).

Between your liver and muscles, you have a ready supply of calories (roughly 300 to 400, depending on your weight and metabolism) that you can access as necessary throughout the day. When you eat more than you can save in these temporary deposits, the calories get converted to fat and stowed throughout your body.

To lose a pound, you have to burn about 3,500 calories. That means you can eat 100 fewer calories a day for 35 days, or 500 fewer calories for 7 days, or walk an hour a day for 22 days, or do a combination of these by eating less and moving more. Remember, even if you're exercising more than usual, the calories-in, calories-out rule still applies: If you take in more than you burn, you'll gain weight.

The Naked Fitness Nutrition Plan automatically controls and modifies your calories for you. You'll be eating between 1,200 and 1,800 calories a day for steady weight loss. Men will be consuming the higher range (1,800) and women, the lower range (1,200).

Eat Breakfast, Burn Fat

"Do I have to eat breakfast even if I'm not hungry?"

I have been asked this question hundreds of times. Here is what I answer: Breakfast is truly the most important meal of the day. Skipping it leads to food cravings later on, intense hunger, and low energy. What's more, research demonstrates that people who regularly eat breakfast keep their weight off; people who don't tend to regain their weight and stay heavy. Eating breakfast is a habit characteristic to maintainers and is a factor in their success.

If you're not in the habit of eating breakfast, force yourself to do so! Eventually you'll get used to a big breakfast—and even look forward to it.

Supplement for Success

Another important benefit of the Naked Fitness Nutrition Plan is that you do not have to spend a lot of extra money on special foods like you would for many other diets. You can buy everything you need at your supermarket. But because you will be consuming fewer calories each day, it is a good idea to supplement your diet with an all-purpose multi-vitamin and mineral supplement that contains antioxidants to prevent any nutrient shortfalls. Antioxidants are vitamins and minerals such as vitamin A, beta-carotene, vitamin C, vitamin E, and selenium that help protect you against disease.

NAKED FITNESS FAT-BURNING PRINCIPLES AT A GLANCE

- A plan providing roughly 30 percent protein, 40 percent carbohydrates, and 30 percent fat promotes significant and effective fat loss.

- Higher amounts of dietary protein result in a greater loss of body fat, with a negligible loss of muscle tissue.

- A reduced amount of carbohydrates provides greater insulin control, so less food is converted to body fat.

- High-fiber foods control appetite and help prevent excess calories from being stored as fat.

- Moderate fat in the diet results in greater weight loss than low-fat diets do.

Add to this a glucosamine-chondroitin supplement. As you age, joint pain and fatigue become growing problems. They prevent people from exercising, and that's a huge barrier to weight loss.

I don't want anything to come between you and an active lifestyle, so I always recommend that people supplement their diets with glucosamine and chondroitin. Both are natural building blocks used to repair connective tissue such as cartilage, tendons, and ligaments.

Found primarily in joint cartilage, glucosamine is a combination of the amino acid glutamine and the sugar glucose. When you take glucosamine, your body incorporates it into molecules called proteoglycans, which help protect your joints and repair damaged cartilage. Research suggests that glucosamine may stimulate cartilage-producing cells known as chondrocytes to build new cartilage, alleviating the symptoms of joint wear and tear.

Studies over the past 25-plus years confirm glucosamine's effectiveness at reducing joint pain. A recent study indicated that it was as effective as ibuprofen for relieving knee osteoarthritis symptoms—good news, as ibuprofen and similar nonsteroidal anti-inflammatory drugs (NSAIDs) have been shown to inhibit muscle growth.

Glucosamine is an effective natural supplement for treating arthritis. A five-year study, published in *Arthritis & Rheumatism* in 2003, showed that patients who took glucosamine experienced less pain, required less medication, and needed fewer joint surgeries. The glucosamine significantly slowed, and sometimes stopped, the progression of the disease.

Chondroitin has the unique ability to distract enzymes bent on destroying cartilage, causing them to target the chondroitin instead. The chondroitin that gets chewed up is then converted to ordinary glucosamine and used to heal joints and tendons.

My favorite form of glucosamine and chondroitin is the kind that comes as a liquid juice-like supplement that's available in pharmacies and grocery stores. The suggested usage of these products in the Naked Fitness Nutrition Plan is one bottle a day at breakfast. It is very delicious, and I take it every day.

Please note that glucosamine is derived from shellfish and chondroitin comes from bovine trachea or pork by-products. There is also a vegan form of glucosamine, so check the labels.

Stay Active for Life

The most effective tool for achieving and maintaining a healthy weight is regular exercise. Not only does it burn energy (calories) and keep your metabolism running in high gear, but it also enhances your self-image— how you feel about yourself. As you experience positive changes in your figure through exercise, you'll begin to feel better about your body and your appearance, both of which contribute to your self-image in a big way. A strong self-image is vital to weight maintenance, and research bears this out. People who frequently relapse and regain their weight have very weak self-images. They see themselves as heavy or ugly and are generally dissatisfied with their bodies. The point is, you can use exercise to prop up your self-image and in doing so, stay the course in keeping your weight off for good.

Exercise helps you maintain your weight loss in other ways too. When you exercise:

- You worry less about your diet and the foods you eat.

- You eat more fruits, vegetables, and other healthy foods, because you want to put high-quality nutrition in your body.

- You feel less depressed and anxious—and less apt to overeat emotionally—because exercise increases mood-elevating chemicals in your body.

- You keep your body toned and trim.

- You like yourself better and tend to treat yourself with greater self-respect—two psychological benefits that fortify you mentally against possible relapses.

Various research studies have calculated the amount of physical activity required to maintain your weight loss. One group of studies reports that women can successfully maintain their weight loss by burning 2,545 calories a week through exercise. That is the equivalent of one hour of brisk walking every day.

The important factor is that you stay physically active. Very few people can maintain their weight loss unless they exercise.

Monitor Your Weight

As you lose weight, it will be vital for you to detect any weight regain in its early stages so you can take action immediately to reverse the trend and avoid a major relapse. There are two ways to accomplish this, and you should use both in conjunction with each other.

First, monitor your weight on a regular basis simply by weighing yourself on your bathroom scale. Research tells us that people who maintain their weight loss frequently monitor their weight this way. In fact, many people weigh themselves as often as once a day; others, just once a week. Regardless of whether you do this daily or weekly, you should make it a point to weigh yourself regularly.

Second, wear clothing that fits you fairly closely (as opposed to baggy outfits) so that you are always aware of your body and tuned in to whether you are regaining any weight. If an article of clothing starts to feel too tight, then that's a signal for you to get back on the "weight-losing track." In a similar vein, periodically try on your bikini or your two-piece bathing suit during the winter and fall months to make sure that it still fits well. Monitoring yourself by using your scale and being aware of your clothes gives you conscious control over the management of your weight.

The Slim Payoff

With the Naked Fitness Nutrition Plan, you're sure to melt away the pounds. The foods you eat will be more satisfying and nutritionally rewarding and will provide the metabolic catalyst you need to shed surplus fat. What exactly are those foods? Keep turning the pages to find out.

8

NAKED FITNESS FOODS

I'll bet the last time you tried to diet, you made sweeping resolutions like "I'm swearing off carbs for good. I will buy only fat free. I'll never drink alcohol. I will give up sweets forever."

We all start with lofty goals, and we all learn the hard way that all-or-nothing diets are very hard to live with over time. Fortunately, on the Naked Fitness Nutrition Plan, you don't have to change your life to change your body. In fact, most experts agree that small modifications, not radical ones, are the key to long-lasting weight loss.

What you'll eat on this program will have a powerful effect on how you look and feel. When I created this program, I wanted to include key foods that are especially helpful if you want to be at your naked best. My food picks can help you achieve three important goals: a healthy weight, increased energy, and radiant health.

Of course, we all know that no single food is a miracle cure. But if you eat a well-balanced diet that emphasizes a variety of foods from my Naked Fitness food list, a few strategic choices can put you over the top in terms of how you look and feel.

Are you ready to give it a try? Over the next two chapters, I'll take you through the foods and menus and show you how to lose pounds and keep them off.

Here comes exactly what you need right now to start losing excess weight and getting in superb shape. As long as you follow my plan to the letter, it will work. If for some reason you discover that you are not losing weight at a reasonable pace, review what you're doing and make sure you aren't deviating from the diet.

So let's get started and look at exactly what you get to eat.

The Naked Fitness Food Groups

Foods in the Naked Fitness Nutrition Plan are organized into six major food groups:

- Fibrous vegetables
- Fruits
- Light proteins
- Calcium-rich proteins
- Starches
- Beneficial fats

If you remember these food groups and what goes into them, it will be easy to plan your meals each day.

Here are the details, including how much to eat from these food groups each day.

Fibrous Vegetables—Unlimited Servings

The Naked Fitness nutrition program places a high priority on fiber-rich vegetables. Any vegetable can be included in your daily diet. Vegetables may be raw or cooked; fresh, frozen, canned, or dried/dehydrated; whole, cut-up, or mashed.

Here is a list of fibrous vegetables you may eat—and in unlimited quantities:

Dark Green Vegetables
Bok choy
Broccoli
Collard greens
Dark green leafy lettuce
Kale
Mustard greens
Romaine lettuce
Spinach
Turnip greens
Watercress

Orange Vegetables
Acorn squash
Butternut squash
Carrots
Hubbard squash
Spaghetti squash

Other Vegetables
Artichokes
Asparagus
Bean sprouts
Beets
Brussels sprouts
Cabbage
Cauliflower
Celery
Cucumbers
Eggplant
Garlic
Green beans
Green, yellow, and red peppers
Iceberg (head) lettuce
Mushrooms
Okra
Onions
Parsnips
Tomatoes
Turnips
Wax beans
Zucchini

HEALTH BENEFITS OF FIBROUS VEGETABLES
If you eat lots of vegetables (fruits too) as part of your overall diet, you protect yourself against an array of chronic diseases. Most vegetables are naturally low in fat and calories. None have cholesterol. (Sauces or seasonings can add fat, calories, or cholesterol.)

Vegetables are important sources of many nutrients, including potassium, dietary fiber, folate (folic acid), vitamin A, beta-carotene, vitamin E, and vitamin C.

Diets rich in potassium may help maintain healthy blood pressure. Vegetable sources of potassium include tomatoes, beet greens, winter squash, and spinach. Dietary fiber from vegetables, as part of an overall healthy diet, helps reduce blood cholesterol levels and may lower the risk of heart disease.

Vitamin A keeps eyes and skin healthy and helps protect against infections. Vitamin E helps protect vitamin A and essential fatty acids from cell oxidation. Vitamin C helps heal cuts and wounds and keeps teeth and gums healthy. Vitamin C also aids in iron absorption.

Vegetables are also rich in plant chemicals called flavonoids. They act as antioxidants that fight free radicals, which are unstable oxygen molecules that attack bodily tissues. Left unchecked, free radicals can cause life-shortening diseases including cancer.

If you eat a diet packed with vegetables:

- You may reduce your risk for stroke and perhaps other cardiovascular diseases, as well as type 2 diabetes.

- You may protect yourself against certain cancers, such as mouth, stomach, and colorectal cancer.

- You may reduce your risk of developing kidney stones and osteoporosis.

- You will keep your weight under control. Eating foods such as vegetables that are low in calories instead of higher-calorie food helps you lower your calorie intake.

SNEAK MORE FIBROUS VEGETABLES INTO YOUR DIET

From working with many people, I know it is challenging to include more veggies in your diet. Here are some suggestions to help you:

- Season your foods with chopped garlic or onion.

- Eat a salad every day.

- Try a new vegetable each week.

- Include at least two vegetables with lunch and dinner.

- Double your portions of vegetables at lunch or dinner.

- Add extra veggies to soups and stews.

- Prepare veggie platters to take to parties.

- When eating out, order sandwiches prepared with tomato, onions, sprouts, peppers, and lettuce.

- At restaurants, choose vegetarian options more often.

- Snack on fresh veggies.

- Vary your veggie choices to keep meals interesting.

- Grill vegetable kabobs as part of a barbecue meal. Try tomatoes, mushrooms, green peppers, and onions.

- Try a low-fat salad dressing with raw broccoli, red and green peppers, celery sticks, or cauliflower.

- Add color to salads by adding baby carrots, shredded red cabbage, or spinach leaves.

- Add pepper to your meal to aid in digestion and add flavor. Skip the salt.

Fruits—Two to Four Servings Daily

Any fruit counts as part of the fruit group on the Naked Fitness Nutrition Plan. Fruits should be eaten fresh. The fruits you may eat include the following:

Apples	Guava	Papaya
Apricots	Honeydew melon	Pineapple
Bananas	Kiwi fruit	Plums
Blackberries	Lemons	Prunes
Blueberries	Limes	Raspberries
Cantaloupe	Mangoes	Strawberries
Cherries	Nectarines	Tangerines
Cranberries	Oranges	Watermelon
Grapefruit	Peaches	Any fruit, as long as
Grapes	Pears	it is fresh

HEALTH BENEFITS OF FRUIT

Eating a diet rich in fruits may reduce your risk of stroke and per-haps other cardiovascular diseases, as well as type 2 diabetes. Fruit also protects you against certain cancers such as mouth, stomach, and colo-rectal cancer.

Fruits are important sources of many nutrients, including potassium, fiber, vitamin C, and folate (folic acid). As I mentioned, diets rich in potas-sium may help maintain healthy blood pressure. Fruit sources of potassium include bananas, prunes and prune juice, dried peaches and apricots, cantaloupe, honeydew melon, and orange juice. Vitamin C is important for growth and repair of all body tissues, helps heal cuts and wounds, and keeps teeth and gums healthy. Fiber-containing foods such as fruits help provide a feeling of fullness with fewer calories. Whole or cut-up fruits are sources of dietary fiber; fruit juices contain little or no fiber.

Folate helps your body form red blood cells. Women of childbearing age who may become pregnant and those in the first trimester of preg-nancy should consume adequate folate, including folic acid from fortified foods or supplements. This reduces the risk of certain birth defects.

To get the most health benefits from fruit:

- Frequently select fruits that are high in potassium such as bananas, prunes and prune juice, dried peaches and apricots, cantaloupe, and honeydew melon.

- Vary your fruit choices. Fruits differ in nutrient content.

- Keep a bowl of whole fruit on the table, on the counter, or in the refrigerator.

- Refrigerate cut-up fruit to store for later.

- Buy fresh fruits in season when they may be less expensive and at their peak flavor.

- Buy fruits that are dried, frozen, and canned (in water or juice) as well as fresh, so that you always have a supply on hand.

- Consider convenience when shopping. Buy packages of precut fruit (such as melon or pineapple chunks) for a healthy snack that's ready in seconds. Choose packaged fruits that do not have added sugars.

- At lunch, pack a tangerine, banana, or grapes or choose fruits from a salad bar. Individual containers of fruits like peaches or pears are easy and convenient.

- Add fruit like pineapple or peaches to kabobs as part of a barbecue meal.

- For dessert, have baked apples, pears, or a fruit salad.

Light Proteins—Three Servings Daily

Foods such as meat, poultry, fish, shellfish, and eggs are considered proteins. Most meat and poultry choices should be lean or low fat. Fish contains healthy oils, so choose it frequently instead of meat or poultry. The light proteins you may eat on the Naked Fitness Nutrition Plan include the following:

Meats
Lean cuts of:
  Beef
  Ham
  Lamb
  Pork
  Veal
Game meats:
  Bison
  Rabbit
  Venison
Lean ground meats:
  Beef
  Lamb
  Pork

Poultry
  Chicken
  Turkey
  Ground chicken
  Ground turkey

Eggs
  Chicken eggs
  Duck eggs

Fish
Finfish:
  Catfish
  Cod
  Flounder
  Haddock
  Halibut
  Herring
  Mackerel
  Pollock
  Salmon
  Sea bass
  Snapper
  Swordfish
  Tilapia
  Trout
  Tuna

Shellfish:
  Clams
  Crab
  Crawfish
  Lobster
  Mussels
  Octopus
  Oysters
  Scallops
  Squid (calamari)
  Shrimp

Canned fish
  packed in water
  or mustard
  (no oil):
Anchovies
Clams
Salmon
Sardines
Tuna

CHOOSING WISELY

When choosing proteins, watch out for those high in saturated fats such as fatty cuts of beef, pork, and lamb; regular (75% to 85% lean) ground beef; regular sausages, hot dogs, and bacon; some luncheon meats such as regular bologna and salami; and some poultry such as duck. Diets high in these fats raise bad cholesterol levels in the blood. The bad cholesterol is called LDL (low-density lipoprotein) cholesterol. High LDL cholesterol increases the risk of coronary heart disease. To help keep blood cholesterol levels healthy, avoid these foods. Diets that are high in cholesterol can raise LDL cholesterol levels in the blood. A high intake of fats makes it difficult to avoid consuming more calories than are needed. If you are unsure of cholesterol levels in meats, use this simple rule of thumb: If the animal is lean and fast while alive, it will typically be very lean and lower in cholesterol when consumed. If an animal is slow and heavy while alive, it will typically be higher in fat and cholesterol when consumed. (Eat fast food!)

VARY YOUR PROTEIN SELECTIONS

Many people do not make varied enough choices from the light protein group, selecting meat or poultry every day as their main dishes. Varying choices and including fish in meals can boost your intake of mono-unsaturated fatty acids and polyunsaturated fatty acids (PUFAs). Most fat in the diet should come from these fats.

Some fish (such as salmon, trout, and herring) are packed with omega-3 fatty acids, which have a wide range of benefits, from protecting the heart to counteracting the effects of aging.

Here are some tips to help you go lean with protein:

- Know the lean choices: The leanest beef cuts include round steaks and roasts (round eye, top round, bottom round, round tip), top loin, top sirloin, and chuck shoulder and leg roasts. The leanest pork choices include pork loin, tenderloin, center loin, and ham.

- Choose extra-lean ground beef. The label should say at least "90% lean." You may be able to find ground beef that is 93% or 95% lean.

- Buy skinless chicken parts or remove the skin before cooking.

- Boneless skinless chicken breasts and turkey cutlets are the leanest poultry choices.

- Choose lean turkey, roast beef, ham, or low-fat luncheon meats for sandwiches instead of luncheon meats with more fat such as regular bologna or salami.

- Trim away all of the visible fat from meats and poultry before cooking.

- Broil, grill, roast, poach, or boil meat, poultry, and fish instead of frying.

- Drain off any fat that appears during cooking.

- Skip or limit the breading on meat, poultry, and fish. Breading adds fat and calories. It will also cause the food to soak up more fat during frying.

- Choose and prepare foods without high-fat sauces or gravies.

- Every day, eat protein with each of your three main meals—breakfast, lunch, and dinner.

- Consider cholesterol. Did you know that the faster and more active the animal while alive, the lower the cholesterol in that animal? As noted previously, how active an animal is while alive determines the animal's fat and cholesterol levels when consumed. Chickens and turkeys are faster and more active than cows and pigs, for example, and therefore lower in cholesterol. The same is true for certain shell-fish: Shrimp and salmon are more active than scallops and lobsters. This is an easy way to make lower-cholesterol choices.

A serving of protein is:

- Four to eight ounces of meat, fish, or poultry
- Three eggs

Eggs are an important part of this food group and deserve honorable mention. Eating eggs instead of bagels for breakfast can help you lose more weight. A recent study found that people who ate two eggs for breakfast lost 65 percent more weight, even though they ate the same number of calories for breakfast. In addition, the egg eaters lost more body fat and had higher energy levels throughout the day, with no change in cholesterol levels.

Calcium-Rich Proteins—One to Two Servings Daily

The Naked Fitness Nutrition Plan also includes certain calcium-rich proteins, including Greek-style yogurt, kefir, cottage cheese, and protein-enriched milk (my favorite is Muscle Milk Light).

I really like to see people eat more yogurt. Yogurt is rich in calcium, which can enhance your body's fat-burning mechanisms. In one study, people who ate three servings of fat-free yogurt lost 22 percent more weight and 61 percent more body fat than people who just cut calories without increasing calcium intake. Yogurt eaters also lost more weight in the hard-to-slim abdominal area while maintaining lean muscle mass.

HEALTH BENEFITS

Diets rich in calcium help build and maintain bone mass throughout the lifecycle. This may reduce the risk of osteoporosis. Diets that include dairy products tend to have a higher overall nutritional quality because they are high in calcium, potassium, and vitamin D, among other nutrients.

The body uses calcium for building bones and teeth and in maintaining bone mass. Dairy products are the primary source of calcium in American diets. Dairy products are also rich in potassium, which may help to maintain healthy blood pressure.

Vitamin D functions to maintain proper levels of calcium and phosphorous, thereby helping build and maintain bones. Dairy products that are fortified with vitamin D are a good source of this nutrient.

FAT-BURNING AND CALCIUM-RICH FOODS

While it does your body and bones good, these foods are also doing good for your figure by helping you lose weight, shed belly fat, and maintain your weight loss. Intake of calcium, especially from dairy products, may influence how the body metabolizes energy according to a growing body of research into this amazing mineral.

A University of Tennessee study found that when obese African American men increased their daily calcium intakes from 400 milligrams to 1,000 milligrams, they had a drop in body fat without a significant change in body weight. This suggests a role for calcium in reducing obesity. Researchers believe that dietary calcium appears to shift energy use from storage in fat to oxidation in muscle. Previous clinical studies have shown that calcium-rich foods enhance weight control and prevent weight regain. A research team from Baylor College of Medicine and Texas Woman's University in Houston reported an association between the consumption of low-fat milk and dairy products and slimmer waists.

Supplements appear to work too. In a 2009 study described in the *British Journal of Nutrition*, obese women who followed a low-calorie diet and took 1,200 milligrams of a daily calcium supplement lost about 13 pounds in 15 weeks, compared to an average loss of 2.2 pounds for women who followed the same diet but took a placebo.

Here are some suggestions for harnessing the fat-burning power of these foods:

- Have fat-free or low-fat yogurt as a snack.
- Make a yogurt dip for fruits or vegetables.
- Make fruit and yogurt smoothies in the blender.
- Top cut-up fruit with flavored yogurt for a quick dessert.
- Top a baked potato with fat-free or low-fat yogurt.

Serving sizes are as follows:

- A six-ounce carton of Greek-style yogurt, which tends to be higher in protein than conventional yogurts. But always check the labels for protein content, since even some so-called Greek yogurts are not high in protein.
- One cup kefir (a fermented milk drink that contains several major strains of friendly bacteria not commonly found in yogurt)
- One low-fat cup cottage cheese
- A 14-ounce container of protein-enriched milk

Starches—Zero to Three Servings Daily

Starches are carbohydrates that are high in fat-fighting fiber, as well as various vitamins and minerals. The starches on the Naked Fitness Nutrition Plan have been specifically selected because they do not stimulate fat storage by causing tremendous swings in insulin and blood sugar. The foods you may eat from this group include, barley, low-carb tortillas, corn, potatoes, and beans and legumes.

Here is a detailed list:

Grain-Based Starches
Barley
Low-carb tortillas
Quinoa (a high-protein grain)

Vegetable Starches
Corn
Potatoes

Beans and Legumes

Black beans
Black-eyed peas
Chickpeas (garbanzo beans)
Edamame
Kidney beans
Lentils

Lima beans
Navy beans
Pinto beans
Soy beans
Split peas
White beans

Servings are as follows:
- Potato: one medium
- Corn: one cup
- Barley: one cup
- Quinoa: ½ cup
- Legumes: (beans and lentils): ½ cup
- Low-carb tortilla: one

Beneficial Fats—One to Three Servings Daily

The Naked Fitness Nutrition Plan is moderate in fat. The fat you eat generally comes from natural sources such as nuts and salad dressings.

Each day, eat one to three servings of these foods. A serving size is:

- One ounce of walnuts (14 halves)
- One ounce of almonds (about a handful)
- Two tablespoons of salad dressing, any type (preferably low-fat)

What About Snacks?

I strongly recommend that you incorporate snacks into your meal planning, at least one or two a day to help keep your metabolism elevated. Keeping your daily allotment of various foods in mind, you can plan snacks in the following manner:

- Fruit servings (if not used with one of your regular meals)
- One serving of calcium-rich food (if not used with one of your regular meals)
- One ounce of walnuts or almonds
- One ounce of trail mix
- Two ounces of a protein
- Fibrous vegetables
- Any combination of the above foods (for example: one cup of nonfat yogurt with one cup of berries)

Portion Control

People who successfully maintain their weight over the long term practice portion control, and you'll do the same.

This requires that you continue to eat controlled quantities of food, as designated by the plan, and avoid taking second helpings. Be aware of what constitutes a serving and don't fudge it by taking more than is

NAKED FITNESS NUTRITION PLAN SERVING SIZES

Food Group	Serving Size
Light proteins— 3 servings daily	4 to 8 oz. cooked lean meat, poultry, or fish; 3 eggs
Calcium-rich proteins— 1 to 3 servings daily	6 oz. carton Greek-style yogurt, 1 cup kefir, 1 cup cottage cheese, 14 oz. protein-enriched milk
Starches— 0 to 3 servings daily	1 cup cooked barley, 1 low-carb tortilla, ½ cup cooked beans or legumes, 1 potato
Fibrous vegetables— unlimited	½ cup cooked or chopped raw vegetables, 1 cup raw, leafy vegetables
Fruit— 2 to 4 servings daily	1 medium piece of raw fruit, ½ grapefruit, 1 melon wedge, 1 cup berries
Beneficial fats— 1 to 3 servings daily	2 tablespoons low-fat salad dressing; 1 oz. (14 halves) walnuts; 1 oz. almonds (20–30 nuts); 1 oz. trail mix (handful)

allotted. Serving sizes for the Naked Fitness Nutrition Plan are listed in the chart above.

Fluids and Beverages for Fat Loss

Drink up for weight loss! That's right. Drinking more water can indirectly help you stay lean. Your kidneys need water to do their job of filtering waste products from the body. If they don't get enough water, the kidneys need backup, so they turn to the liver for help. One of the liver's many functions is mobilizing stored fat for energy. When it takes on extra work from the kidneys, the liver can't do its fat-burning job as well. Fat loss is compromised as a result, so you have to drink enough water to keep your body's fat-burning processes proceeding full steam ahead.

Water is vital for other reasons. It accounts for one-half to four-fifths of your weight and performs countless vital chores in the body. It provides the medium in which life-sustaining chemical reactions take place. Water also serves as a solvent for minerals, vitamins, amino acids, glucose, and many other nutrients. Without water, you can't even digest these essential nutrients, let alone absorb, transport, and utilize them. When your temperature rises, water is to your body what coolant is to the radiator of your car. Water is so essential that you'll die within a week without it.

The amount of water you need for good health varies, depending partly on your activity level. On average, you should drink a minimum of eight to ten cups of water every day if you're not active. Since you'll be exercising, you need this minimum, but it's also a good idea to replace the fluids lost during exercise.

You can easily tell if you're not getting enough water by noting the following signs:

- Fatigue
- Loss of appetite
- Flushed skin
- Heat intolerance
- Light-headedness
- Dark urine with a strong odor

Today you can have spring water, mineral water, tap water, and sparkling water, and the list goes on. With so many choices, which one's for you?

The most convenient choice is tap water straight from your faucet. Tap water contains a variety of minerals. In most cities, it's chlorinated and fluoridated. The mineral content in tap water varies regionally, and the amount of chlorine and fluoride added to water is regulated.

Bottled water is generally a better choice than tap water because of possible contamination of tap water. Tap water in many areas contains contaminants such as pesticides, chlorine by-products, and harmful microorganisms. If you drink tap water, a good move is to buy a water purifier, which filters out some contaminants. No matter what kind of water you choose, the bottom line is to drink lots of it.

In the next chapter, I'll show you how to take the foods from my six food groups and turn them into delicious, satisfying fat-burning meals.

ITEMS TO KEEP ON HAND
IN THE NAKED FITNESS KITCHEN

- Greek yogurt with a minimum of 13 grams of protein per 1 cup serving
- Fresh leafy greens like spinach or romaine lettuce
- A bunch of bananas
- Apples
- Extra-virgin olive oil
- Lean turkey or chicken lunchmeat
- Low-carbohydrate tortillas
- Black beans and kidney beans
- Tuna (3-ounce packs of premium albacore)
- Berries, fresh or frozen
- Bag of almonds or walnuts (I keep these in the freezer)
- Green tea
- At least one lemon and lime (add to water or salads)
- At least four chicken breasts (buy in bulk, grill on the weekends, and freeze some)

ITEMS TO KEEP ON HAND
IN THE NAKED FITNESS KITCHEN (continued)

- Peppers (I try to keep at least one red and green in the fridge)
- Frozen broccoli (to add to any meal)
- A dozen large eggs
- Smart Snackin Gourmet Meat Snacks (50 calories; combine with a piece of fruit for a great snack)
- Muscle Milk Light chocolate flavor (100 calories)
- Morning Star Tomato & Basil Veggie Burger (120 calories; add a grilled portobello mushroom for a bun and a splash of low-fat dressing)
- Morning Star Spicy Black Bean Burger (120 calories)
- Trader Joe's Mahi Mahi Burger (110 calories)
- Trader Joe's Roast Florentine (240 calories)
- Pepper for seasoning
- Organic lowfat kefir raspberry (174 calories a cup)
- Raisin River Sweet Italian Chicken Sausage (176 calories 16 grams protein)

9

THE NAKED FITNESS MEAL PLANS

Now let's put everything together, with exactly what you need right now to start losing excess weight and getting in superb shape. In this chapter we'll describe the Naked Fitness meal plans. They're doable and fun. As long as you follow them closely, they will work. So let's get started.

Following the Program

The Naked Fitness meal plans incorporate all of the fat-burning nutrition principles described in the previous chapter. On average, the plan supplies approximately 1,200 to 1,800 calories a day. Usually no more than 30 percent of those calories come from fat.

Men, please note: In each of the six food groups, choose the higher number of servings. For example, the number of servings for starches is zero to three daily. If you are a man, eat three servings of starches each day.

Remember too that this plan is high in protein while providing moderate amounts of carbohydrates—two dietary strategies that encourage fat loss. This balance of protein and carbohydrates helps control hormones (less insulin production) in favor of fat loss.

Featuring 28 days of meals, the program is not a rigid diet but rather a guide for how to eat healthfully every day. At first, you might want to follow the plan exactly. Then, as you get the hang of it, you can adapt it to your own food preferences.

Feel free to swap meals whenever you wish. You can eat a Day 1 or Day 2 breakfast every day of the week, have a Day 16 lunch on Day 5, and so forth. This program is very flexible and is designed to be a guide for you on your way to a beautiful naked body.

You can find a number of my delicious recipes in Appendix F. I've also included grocery lists for each week to make everything even easier. For special diets (kosher, vegan, gluten-free, etc.) visit www .nakedfitness.com

Eat well and enjoy!

Week One

Here is the shopping list and menu plan for you to follow for the first week. It's not hard to follow; no meal takes more than 15 minutes to make. If you add in your walking every day, you may find some extra room in your pants by the end of the week. Get started today and start eating healthier!

GROCERY LIST FOR WEEK ONE
Fibrous Vegetables
3 cups asparagus, fresh or approximately 3 bundles
5 cups broccoli, chopped, fresh approximately 5 heads
4 cups green beans (snap) (approximately 2 pounds)
About 16 cups romaine lettuce, fresh spinach, or mixed greens (approximately 4 bags)
3 cups red pepper, chopped (2 large or 3 medium)
4 cups spinach, fresh (about 4 oz.) approximately 2 bags
20 cherry tomatoes (approximately 1 pint)

Fresh Fruits

6 medium gala apples (2¾-inch diameter) (approximately 3 per pound)

7 firm medium bananas (7 to 7⅞ inches long)

3 cups blueberries, fresh or frozen, unsweetened approximately 2.5 pints

2 cups raspberries approximately 2 pints

Light Proteins

Approximately 2 lbs. chicken breast, no skin

Chicken sausage (Trader Joe's Spicy Jalapeno or similar flavor), one 12-oz. package

6 oz. cod (fish)

12 oz. filet mignon (two 6-oz. filets)

2 oz. ham, extra lean (5% fat)

9 large eggs, fresh

Calcium-Rich Proteins

5 cups Greek yogurt, nonfat plain, (Fage 0%) 40 oz.

Six 6-oz. containers Greek yogurt, nonfat with fruit (Chobani), (140 calories, 12 to 18 grams protein)

Starches

One 15-oz. can chickpeas (garbanzo beans)

One 18-oz. tube polenta (prepared)

Beneficial Fats

3 oz. walnuts

Kraft Light Done Right Zesty Italian Salad Dressing or other dressing where 2 tbsp. contains less than 50 calories and less than 4.5 grams of fat

Frozen Foods

2 cups edamame, shelled, frozen

Spices/Herbs/Condiments/Sauces

One 12-oz. tub salsa (under 125 calories for entire tub; I recommend fresh salsa)

Supplements
Liquid glucosamine supplement, 1 serving per day (has joint supplements
    and calcium for weight loss)

WEEK 1, DAY 1
Breakfast
Blueberries, 1 cup
Greek yogurt, plain nonfat, 1 carton (6 oz.)
Walnuts, 1 oz. (14 halves)
Liquid glucosamine supplement, 1 serving

Lunch
Chicken breast, no skin, 6 oz.
Romaine lettuce (salad), 3 cups shredded
Red pepper, ½ large
Salad dressing, low-fat, 2 tbsp.

Dinner
Chicken breast, no skin, 6 oz.
Green beans (snap), 1 cup
Broccoli, fresh, 1 cup chopped

Snacks
Banana, fresh, 1 medium
Apple, fresh, 1 medium
Greek yogurt, nonfat with fruit, 1 carton (6 oz.)

WEEK 1, DAY 2
Breakfast
Raspberries, 1 cup
Greek yogurt, plain nonfat, 1 carton (6 oz.)
Walnuts, ½ oz. (7 halves)
Liquid glucosamine supplement, 1 serving

Lunch
Naked Fitness polenta chili, 1 serving
Apple, fresh, 1 medium

Dinner
Cod (fish), baked, 6 oz.
Asparagus, fresh, 1 cup
Broccoli, fresh, 1 cup, chopped

Snacks
Banana, fresh, 1 medium
Greek yogurt, plain nonfat, 1 carton (6 oz.)

WEEK 1, DAY 3
Breakfast
Eggs, fresh, 3 large, prepared without oil
Cherry tomatoes, 8
Red pepper, ¼ large
Liquid glucosamine supplement, 1 serving

Lunch
Naked Fitness polenta chili, 1 serving
Red pepper, ¼ large
Romaine lettuce (salad), 3 cups, shredded
Salad dressing, low-fat, 2 tbsp.

Dinner
Chicken breast, no skin, 4 oz.
Green beans (snap), 1 cup
Asparagus, fresh, 1 cup

Snacks
Apple, fresh, 1 medium
Greek yogurt, nonfat, 1 carton (6 oz.)

WEEK 1, DAY 4

Breakfast

Blueberries, 1 cup

Greek yogurt, plain nonfat, 1 carton (6 oz.)

Walnuts, ½ oz. (7 halves)

Liquid glucosamine supplement, 1 serving

Lunch

Naked Fitness polenta chili, 1 serving

Apple, fresh, 1 medium

Dinner

Chicken breast, no skin, 6 oz.

Broccoli, fresh, ½ cup, chopped

Romaine lettuce (salad), 3 cups shredded

Red pepper, ¼ large

Salad dressing, low-fat, 2 tbsp.

Snacks

Apple, fresh, 1 medium

Greek yogurt, plain nonfat, 1 carton (6 oz.)

Banana, fresh, 1 medium

WEEK 1, DAY 5

Breakfast

Eggs, fresh, 3 large, prepared without oil

Asparagus, fresh, ½ cup

Cherry tomatoes, 8

Liquid glucosamine supplement, 1 serving

Lunch
Chicken breast, no skin, 4 oz.
Edamame, shelled, frozen, ½ cup
Romaine lettuce (salad), 3 cups shredded
Red pepper ¼ large
Salad dressing, low-fat, 2 tbsp.

Dinner
Naked Fitness polenta chili, 1 serving
Romaine lettuce (salad), 1 cup shredded
Red pepper, ¼ large
Salad dressing, low-fat, 2 tbsp.

Snacks
Greek yogurt, plain nonfat, 1 carton (6 oz.)
Banana, fresh, 1 medium

WEEK 1, DAY 6
Breakfast
Blueberries, 1 cup
Greek yogurt, plain nonfat, 1 carton (6 oz.)
Walnuts, ½ oz. (7 halves)
Liquid glucosamine supplement, 1 serving

Lunch
Chicken breast, no skin, 4 oz.
Edamame, shelled, frozen, ½ cup
Romaine lettuce (salad), 3 cups shredded
Red pepper, ¼ large
Salad dressing, low-fat, 2 tbsp.

Dinner
Filet mignon, 6 oz.
Broccoli, fresh, 1 cup chopped
Green beans (snap), ½ cup

Snacks
Apple, fresh, 1 medium
Banana, fresh, 1 medium
Greek yogurt, plain nonfat, 1 carton (6 oz.)

WEEK 1, DAY 7
Breakfast
Eggs, fresh, 3 large, prepared without oil
Ham, extra lean, (5% fat), 2 oz.
Spinach, fresh, 2 cups
Cherry tomatoes, 4
Liquid glucosamine supplement, 1 serving

Lunch
Chicken breast, no skin, 4 oz.
Edamame, shelled, frozen, ½ cup
Spinach, fresh, 2 cups
Salad dressing, low-fat, 2 tbsp.

Dinner
Filet mignon, 6 oz.
Broccoli, fresh, 1 cup chopped
Green beans (snap), 1 cup

Snacks
Raspberries, ½ cup
Banana, fresh, 1 medium
Greek yogurt, plain nonfat, 1 carton (6 oz.)

Week Two

Here is the shopping list and menu plan for you to follow for the next week. Note that you may substitute your favorite meals from last week. Feel free to change around the days.

GROCERY LIST FOR WEEK TWO

Fibrous Vegetables

3 cups (1 bunch) asparagus

4 bags fresh spinach (13 cups)

1 bunch broccoli (3 stalks)

1 cup carrots (diced) (small bag of baby carrots)

1 tub cherry tomatoes (24 tomatoes)

2 cups green beans

1 medium onion (1 cup diced)

1 red pepper, medium (about 2¾ inches long, 2½-inch diameter)

Fresh Fruits

3 crisp apples, medium (2¾-inch diameter) (about 3 per pound)

7 firm bananas, medium (7 to 7⅞ inches long)

2 pints blueberries (or raspberries)

Light Protein

Six 6-oz. chicken breasts, no skin (36 oz. total)

Two 6-oz. filet mignon (or other lean meat)

12 oz. sliced ham, extra lean (5% fat)

8 eggs (6 fresh, plus 2 hardboiled)

Starches

One 12-oz. can black beans

1 package corn tortillas (no more than 90 calories for 2; at least 2 grams fiber) (you'll need 8 tortillas)

Beneficial Fats

2 oz. walnuts (28 halves)

Lite salad dressing (your choice; no more than 50 calories for 2 tbsp.)

Spices/Herbs/Condiments/Sauces
One 12- or 16-oz. jar of salsa (no more than 125 calories for the entire jar)
Cumin, chili powder, cilantro, or a fajita spice packet
Chives, fresh or dried
8 cups chicken stock

Calcium-Rich Protein
One 24-oz. carton cottage cheese
6 cups Greek yogurt, plain nonfat
2 cups Greek yogurt, nonfat with fruit

Supplements
Liquid glucosamine supplement, 1 serving

WEEK 2, DAY 1
Breakfast
Eggs, fresh, 3 large, prepared without oil
Ham, 4 oz.
Spinach, fresh, 1 cup
Cherry tomatoes, 4
Liquid glucosamine supplement, 1 serving

Lunch
Chicken breast, no skin, 4 oz.
Spinach, fresh, 2 cups
Salad dressing, 2 tbsp.

Dinner
Filet mignon, 6 oz.
Broccoli, fresh, 1 cup chopped
Green beans, 1 cup

Snacks
Banana
Berries, ½ cup
Greek yogurt, plain nonfat, 1 carton (6 oz.)

WEEK 2, DAY 2
Breakfast
Berries, 1 cup
Greek yogurt, plain nonfat, 1 carton (6 oz.)
Walnuts, ½ oz. (7 halves)
Liquid glucosamine supplement, 1 serving

Lunch
Apple
Naked Fitness tortilla soup, 1 serving

Dinner
Chicken breast, no skin, 6 oz.
Asparagus, fresh, 1 cup
Broccoli, fresh, ½ cup chopped

Snacks
Banana
Egg, hard boiled, 1 large
Ham, 4 oz.

WEEK 2, DAY 3
Breakfast
Asparagus, fresh, 1 cup
Egg, fresh, 3 large, prepared without oil
Cherry tomatoes, 4
Liquid glucosamine supplement, 1 serving

Lunch
Egg, hard boiled, 1 large
Ham, 4 oz.
Spinach, fresh, 2 cups
Cherry tomatoes, 4
Salad dressing, low-fat, 2 tbsp.

Dinner
Chicken breast, no skin, 6 oz.
Green beans, 1 cup
Asparagus, fresh, 1 cup

Snacks
Apple
Banana
Greek yogurt, plain nonfat, 1 carton (6 oz.)

WEEK 2, DAY 4

Breakfast
Cottage cheese, 1 cup
Cherry tomatoes, 4
Fresh chives, 1 tbsp. chopped
Liquid glucosamine supplement, 1 serving

Lunch
Naked Fitness tortilla soup, 1 serving
Apple

Dinner
Chicken breast, no skin, 6 oz.
Spinach, fresh, 2 cups

Snacks

Banana

Berries, 1 cup

Greek yogurt, plain nonfat, 1 carton (6 oz.)

Walnuts, ½ oz. (7 halves)

WEEK 2, DAY 5

Breakfast

Berries, 1 cup

Greek yogurt, plain nonfat, 1 carton (6 oz.)

Walnuts, ½ oz. (7 halves)

Liquid glucosamine supplement, 1 serving

Lunch

Chicken breast, no skin, 4 oz.

Spinach, fresh, 2 cups

Red pepper, ¼

Salad dressing, low-fat, 2 tbsp.

Dinner

Naked Fitness tortilla soup, 1 serving

Red pepper, ¾

Snacks

Banana

Greek yogurt with fruit, 1 carton (6 oz.)

Walnuts, ½ oz. (7 halves)

WEEK 2, DAY 6

Breakfast

Cottage cheese, 1 cup

Cherry tomatoes, 4

Fresh chives, 1 tbsp. chopped

Liquid glucosamine supplement, 1 serving

Lunch
Naked Fitness tortilla soup, 1 serving
Spinach, fresh, 2 cups
Cherry tomatoes, 4
Salad dressing, low-fat, 2 tbsp.

Dinner
Filet mignon, 6 oz.
Broccoli, fresh, 1 cup chopped
Spinach, fresh, 2 cups

Snacks
Banana
Greek yogurt with fruit, 1 carton (6 oz.)

WEEK 2, DAY 7
Breakfast
Cottage cheese, 1 cup
Cherry tomatoes, 4
Fresh chives, 1 tbsp. chopped
Liquid glucosamine supplement, 1 serving

Lunch
Naked Fitness tortilla soup, 1 serving
Apple

Dinner
Chicken breast, no skin, 6 oz.
Spinach, fresh, 2 cups

Snacks
Banana
Greek yogurt with fruit, 1 carton (6 oz.)

Week Three

Here's the shopping list and plan for the next week.

GROCERY LIST FOR WEEK THREE

Fibrous Vegetables

4 cups asparagus (approximately 3 bunches)

2 cups broccoli

1 cup/1 ear corn fresh or frozen

1 bunch green onions (about 6 stalks)

4 red peppers, (about 4 cups chopped)

3 bags (3 hearts each) romaine lettuce

1 cup spinach

1 pint cherry tomatoes

6 Roma tomatoes

zucchini, 2 cups

Fresh Fruits

5 bananas, medium (7 to 7⅞ inches long)

2 oranges, small (2⅜ inch diameter)

1 pint raspberries

2 lbs. strawberries (about 7 cups)

Starches

2 potatoes, small (1¾- to 2½-inch diameter)

1 cup pearled barley

1 can pinto beans

1 can red kidney beans

Low-carbohydrate, high-fiber tortillas (2 servings)

Calcium-Rich Proteins

10 cartons Greek yogurt, plain nonfat

1 cup Parmesan cheese

Light Proteins
2 lbs. chicken breast, no skin
22 oz. beef, top sirloin
6 oz. salmon
24 oz. shrimp
Eggs, fresh, 15 large

Beneficial Fats
Cilantro salad dressing
Kraft Light Done Right Zesty Italian Salad Dressing
2 oz. walnuts (28 halves)

Supplements
Liquid glucosamine supplement, 1 serving per day
14 oz. Muscle Milk Light (chocolate or vanilla)

WEEK 3, DAY 1

Breakfast
Raspberries, 1 cup
Walnuts, ½ oz. (7 halves)
Greek yogurt, plain nonfat, 1 carton (6 oz.)
Liquid glucosamine supplement, 1 serving

Lunch
Beef, top sirloin, 4 oz.
Romaine lettuce, 3 cups shredded
Roma tomatoes, 2 small
Salad dressing, low-fat, 2 tbsp.

Dinner
Shrimp, cooked, 6 oz.
Romaine lettuce, 2 cups shredded
Red pepper, ½
Salad dressing, low-fat, 2 tbsp.
Baked potato, with skin, 1 small
Corn, 1 cup

Snacks
Strawberries, 1 cup sliced
Banana, 1 medium
Greek Yogurt, plain nonfat, 1 carton (6 oz.)

WEEK 3, DAY 2
Breakfast
Eggs, fresh, 3 large
Spinach, fresh, 1 cup
Green onions, 2 stalks, chopped
Tomatoes, 8 cherry
Banana
Liquid glucosamine supplement, 1 serving

Lunch
Beef, top sirloin, 4 oz.
Romaine lettuce, 1 cup shredded
Red pepper, ¼
Red kidney beans, ¼ cup
Low-carbohydrate tortilla, 1

Dinner
Chicken breast, no skin, 8 oz.
Broccoli, 1 cup chopped
Romaine lettuce, 2 cups shredded
Red pepper, ¼
Salad dressing, low-fat, 2 tbsp.

Snacks
Banana
Strawberries, 1 cup sliced
Greek yogurt, plain nonfat, 1 carton (6 oz.)

WEEK 3, DAY 3
Breakfast
Naked Fitness eggs asparagus, 1 serving
Liquid glucosamine supplement, 1 serving

Lunch
Beef, top sirloin, 4 oz.
Romaine lettuce, 1 cup shredded
Red pepper, ¼
Red kidney beans, ¼ cup
Low-carbohydrate tortilla, 1

Dinner
Chicken breast, no skin, 8 oz.
Broccoli, 1 cup chopped
Romaine lettuce, 2 cups shredded
Red pepper, ¼
Salad dressing, low-fat, 2 tbsp.

Snacks
Strawberries, 1 cup sliced
Greek yogurt, plain nonfat, 1 carton (6 oz.)
Orange, 1 small

WEEK 3, DAY 4
Breakfast
Strawberries, 1 cup
Walnuts, ½ oz. (7 halves)
Greek yogurt, plain nonfat, 1 carton (6 oz.)
Liquid glucosamine supplement, 1 serving

Lunch
Shrimp, 6 oz.
Romaine lettuce, 2 cups shredded
Red pepper, ¼
Cilantro salad dressing, 2 tbsp.
Red kidney beans, ½ cup
Pinto beans, ½ cup

Dinner
Salmon, 6 oz.
Asparagus, fresh, 1½ cup
Zucchini, ½ cup, sliced
Barley, pearled, cooked, 1 cup

Snacks
Banana
Greek yogurt, plain nonfat, 1 carton (6 oz.)

WEEK 3, DAY 5
Breakfast
Raspberries, 1 cup
Walnuts, ½ oz. (7 halves)
Greek yogurt, plain nonfat, 1 carton (6 oz.)
Liquid glucosamine supplement, 1 serving

Lunch
Beef, top sirloin, 6 oz.
Romaine lettuce, 3 cups shredded
Roma tomatoes, 2 small
Salad dressing, low-fat, 2 tbsp.

Dinner

Chicken breast, no skin, 8 oz.

Zucchini, ½ cup sliced

Romaine lettuce, 2 cups shredded

Red pepper, ¼

Salad dressing, low-fat, 2 tbsp.

Snacks

Strawberries, 1 cup sliced

Muscle Milk Light (14 oz. bottle), chocolate or vanilla

Greek yogurt, plain nonfat, 1 carton (6 oz.)

WEEK 3, DAY 6

Breakfast

Raspberries, 1 cup

Walnuts, ½ oz. (7 halves)

Greek yogurt, plain nonfat, 1 carton (6 oz.)

Liquid glucosamine supplement, 1 serving

Lunch

Shrimp (boiled or steamed), 6 oz.

Red kidney beans, ½ cup

Pinto beans, ½ cup

Romaine lettuce, 2 cups shredded

Red pepper, ½ cup chopped

Cilantro salad dressing, 2 tbsp.

Dinner

Chicken breast, no skin, 8 oz.

Romaine lettuce, 2 cups shredded

Zucchini, ½ cup sliced

Red pepper, ¼

Salad dressing, low-fat, 2 tbsp.

Snacks
Orange, 1 small
Strawberries, 1 cup sliced
Greek yogurt, plain nonfat, 1 carton (6 oz.)

WEEK 3, DAY 7
Breakfast
Naked Fitness eggs asparagus, 1 serving
Liquid glucosamine supplement, 1 serving

Lunch
Shrimp, 6 oz.
Romaine lettuce, 2 cups shredded
Red pepper, ½ chopped
Cilantro salad dressing, 2 tbsp.
Red kidney beans, ½ cup
Pinto beans, ½ cup

Dinner
Beef, top sirloin, 4 oz.
Baked potato, with skin, 1 small
Romaine lettuce, 2 cups shredded
Red pepper, ¼
Salad dressing, low-fat, 2 tbsp.

Snacks
Banana
Strawberries, 1 cup sliced
Greek yogurt, plain nonfat, 1 carton (6 oz.)

Week Four

This is the first week you're on your own! Now that you've got the hang of the plan, you can begin planning your own meals. Below is a "blueprint" to show you how the Naked Fitness meal plans are structured and to help you with your own meal planning.

THE NAKED FITNESS MEAL BLUEPRINT

BREAKFAST
1 serving fresh fruit
1 light protein or calcium-rich protein
Liquid glucosamine supplement, 1 serving

SNACK
1 to 2 fruits

LUNCH
1 protein serving (4 to 6 oz.)
Fibrous vegetables

DINNER
1 protein serving (6 to 8 oz.)
Fibrous vegetables

OTHER
Add in 0 to 3 starch servings to any part of the menu
Add in 1 to 3 servings of beneficial fats to any part of the menu
Add in 1 to 2 servings of calcium-rich protein to any part of the menu

Simply slot in the foods you'd like to eat, and you're all set. To help you this week, here are a few sample meals.

Sample Breakfasts

- Greek yogurt with 1 cup fresh berries, 1 banana, and 10 almonds
- 3 eggs with 1 cup steamed veggies, 2 oz. cheddar cheese, and tea
- 3 hard boiled eggs, 1 orange, and 1 slice whole-grain bread

TIP: Try getting veggies in the morning with your fruit by cooking twice as many the night before to use the next morning.

Sample Lunches

- Mexico Quickie: ½ cup black beans, 4 oz. chicken breast, ½ cup chopped red pepper, 1 tbsp. vinaigrette, all rolled up in a low-carbohydrate tortilla (21 g fiber)
- 2 cups spinach; ½ cup string beans; ¼ cup each: chopped peppers, onions, carrots, beets, red cabbage; 1 tbsp. balsamic dressing
- Tuna Fast: One 3 oz. package drained tuna, ½ cup red peppers, 2 tbsp. low-carb barbecue sauce over 2 cups mixed greens; slice of watermelon

TIP: Add dark-colored beans to increase the fiber and protein.

Sample Dinners

- Charlie's Tuna: 6 oz. seared tuna, 4 oz. quinoa prepared with chicken broth
- 6 oz. grilled chicken, 2 cups cooked spinach, 1 cup fresh berries with 1 tbsp. sugar-free whipped topping, ¼ cup yogurt, tea
- 1 cup spaghetti squash with 1 tsp. maple syrup, 1 cup mashed cauliflower, 1 cup cooked barley pearls, ¼ cup trail mix, 4 oz. grilled chicken breast, ¼ cup yogurt

Eating Out on the Naked Fitness Nutrition Plan

It's normal to want to get out of the kitchen occasionally and let someone else do the cooking. But what about sticking to the plan? Will dining out strike a fatal blow to your resolve? Not necessarily. Most restaurants cater to health-conscious diners, so it's not that difficult to find low-fat cuisine while dining out.

According to the National Restaurant Association, Americans eat out 4.1 times a week. And many of those meals are eaten at fast-food restaurants, where food is typically high in fat and sodium. But dining out doesn't have to spell dieting disaster. One of the many advantages of the Naked Fitness Nutrition Plan is its adaptability to any eating-out situation. These days, healthy foods are served practically everywhere.

You don't have to be a recluse while on the Naked Fitness Nutrition Plan. You're free to go out to restaurants, even fast-food places, to enjoy breakfast, lunch, or dinner with your friends, family, or business associates. Nor should you pass up invitations to parties or other social events just because you're on a healthy eating program.

What follows are some practical guidelines for making healthy choices at any type of restaurant, as well as for enjoying parties and other events.

Restaurants for Breakfast

- Order scrambled eggs. Request that the eggs be cooked without added oil.

- Fresh fruits are excellent choices to round out your breakfast.

Asian Restaurants

- Select entrees made with lean proteins (such as chicken and fish) and vegetables. Some good suggestions are Moo Goo Gai Pan, Szechwan Shrimp or Chicken, and sushi.

- Request that the sauce be served on the side or forgo it altogether.

- Asian restaurants serve generous helpings. Consider ordering one entree and splitting it with a friend, unless you want to take the leftovers home.
- Enjoy sushi and sashimi.

Italian Restaurants

- For an appetizer, try vegetable antipasto (if available), with dressing on the side.
- Look for entrees such as grilled chicken and fish, as well as Italian dishes that are marked as low in fat.
- Avoid entrees prepared in cream sauce or Alfredo sauce.
- Ask the waiter to leave the rolls and breadsticks in the kitchen.
- When ordering a dinner salad, request dressing on the side.
- Opt for steamed vegetables as your side dish rather than pasta. Make sure the vegetables are steamed.

Mexican Restaurants

- Grilled chicken, shrimp, or lean meat entrees are good choices.
- For extra veggies, request pico de gallo (a mixture of chopped tomatoes, green peppers, and onions).
- Mexican rice or black bean soup are nice accompaniments to a Mexican meal. So are refried beans, but check first to see whether they are prepared in lard, or baked or boiled, and seasoned. If they aren't refried in lard, enjoy them.
- A dinner salad with nonfat salad dressing is a healthy meal-starter.

Steakhouse

- Order grilled lean meat, chicken, salmon, or other fish (prepared without oil).
- For a side dish, select a steamed vegetable such as broccoli.
- At the salad bar, stick to fresh vegetables. Many salad bars serve fresh fruit too, which makes for a great dessert.

Homestyle or Cafeteria Restaurant

- Request grilled or lemon chicken, turkey breast without the gravy, or white fish prepared without sauce or oil.
- Select steamed vegetables (no sauce or butter), salad with nonfat dressing, or a vegetable medley prepared without butter or margarine.
- Look away when passing by the dessert line.

Fast-Food Restaurants

- Most fast-food establishments have salads on their menus; grilled chicken salads are your best bets. Order reduced-fat salad dressing with your salad. If there's a salad bar, stick to fresh vegetables and fat-free salad dressing.
- At fast-food restaurants that serve fish, order baked fish, steamed vegetables, and a salad.

Parties

- Eat a meal before you go to the party to fend off hunger pangs and cravings.
- Snack on fresh vegetables and fruit (but pass up the dip).
- If you're going to dinner with a group of friends and are concerned that you'll overeat, eat some natural high-fiber foods (like raw vegetables or fruit) before you go. You'll be less likely to pig out later.
- Offer to bring a couple of your own dishes (low-fat, of course) to the gathering.
- Instead of a cocktail, drink a diet soda or carbonated water with a twist of lemon or lime.

It may not seem like fun to limit yourself to certain foods when eating out. But the ability to make healthy choices at restaurants is one more positive step toward getting a beautifully naked body. You'll feel better, and your body will love you for it.

Nutritional Boosters

Whether starting the Naked Fitness Nutrition Plan or renewing a commitment to get fit, everyone needs some "booster shots" from time to time to shore up motivation. Toward that end, here are 50 of my best tips for sticking to the plan so that you burn body fat and look great in your naked body.

1. Eat all required foods on the plan: three light proteins, zero to three natural starches, two to four fruits, unlimited fibrous vegetables, one to two calcium-rich proteins, and one to three beneficial fats. Never skip a thing!

2. Use spices and seasonings (low-sugar or sugar-free products) to flavor your foods.

3. Do not drink fruit juices or juice-based products while following the plan. These products are devoid of fiber and will not help you lose surplus fat. Get your nutrition from calories you chew.

4. Shoot for 25 grams of fiber daily. (The Naked Fitness Nutrition Plan incorporates this requirement each day of the week.)

5. If you feel hungry, it's permissible to eat a few ounces of extra protein to tame your appetite and tide you over.

6. Eat at least two servings of fish a week to obtain a type of healthy fat called omega-3 fatty acids. These beneficial fats help your body in numerous ways, including reducing triglycerides (fats in your blood), boosting your aerobic power, and normalizing your mood.

7. Eat very lean meat; remove all visible fat before cooking. Remove skin and fat from poultry before cooking.

8. With the exception of lean and fat-free lunch meats, avoid cured and smoked foods. They're high in fat, salt, and nitrates (which are carcinogens).

9. Choose liberally from the list of fibrous vegetables, especially for salads.

10. Colorize your meals. The more colorful your plate, the healthier your meal is. The key to colorizing your meals is to understand that each fruit or vegetable, whether it's blue, red, or green, is made up of a

different combination of phytochemicals. Phytochemicals are non-nutritive plant substances that have disease-prevention properties and give each piece of produce its color. Each color of food offers different health benefits to the body. Therefore, by consuming a variety of foods in various colors, you'll get the full range of nutrients needed to keep your body healthy and strong.

11. Prepare your salads with your daily fat allotment, with low-fat salad dressings, or vinegar.

12. Spice your foods with red pepper (capsicum). This popular seasoning is believed to rev up your metabolism by creating heat. You've probably noticed this yourself. After you eat hot spicy foods, your body will heat up in a process known as "diet-induced thermogenesis." When body temperature rises, so does metabolism, and you burn more calories.

13. Blend nonfat yogurt with low-fat cottage cheese for vegetable dips.

14. Drizzle sugar-free syrup over cooked carrots for a sweet treat.

15. Try using lemon juice or various herbs on your vegetables, rather than eating them with too much added fat.

16. Do not substitute or add to the Naked Fitness Nutrition Plan.

17. Avoid alcoholic beverages while trying to lose body fat. Excessive consumption of alcohol strains your liver, which responds by slowing down functions like fat burning and waste elimination. A liver that's on the edge throws a monkey wrench into weight loss. Have a sparkling no-calorie beverage with a twist of lemon or lime when you're out.

18. In addition to water, you may drink the following beverages: regular or decaffeinated tea, green tea, herbal teas, regular or decaffeinated coffee, carbonated water, and mineral water.

19. Write down what you will eat each day for better control over your food intake. Use the worksheet provided in Appendix I.

20. Drizzle balsamic vinegar over cooked vegetables for tangy flavor.

21. When you snack, choose foods from your calcium-rich proteins, fibrous vegetables, fruits, and fats such as nuts.

22. Drink eight to ten glasses of water a day. Water aids in weight loss by dulling your appetite and enhancing fat-burning processes in your body.

23. Drink green tea liberally; it can be helpful in burning fat.

24. Take a good-quality vitamin and mineral supplement each day.

25. Do not overeat.

26. Don't skip meals. Skipping meals only makes you hungry later.

27. Slow down your eating and chew your food thoroughly. Both actions help you feel full faster and are a proven weight-control tactic.

28. Do you overeat or oversnack in front of the television? If so, make it a rule in your house to always eat in the dining room, seated at the table.

29. Try not to let yourself get bored, stressed out, or depressed. For help on this, see Chapter 14.

30. Do you like to nibble in the kitchen while fixing dinner? The calories in those extra bites can really add up. Chew some sugarless gum, sip water, or keep low-calorie snacks such as raw veggies on hand while you're cooking. If you don't have time to cut up vegetables, buy precut veggies (or fruits) from the grocery store or take advantage of the store's salad bar, which usually has plenty of freshly cut items.

31. Outwait your food cravings. They generally last no longer than 10 minutes. If you feel the urge to splurge, find something else to do for 10 minutes or until the craving passes.

32. Be assertive when people offer you food. Train yourself to say "No, thank you."

33. Visualize what you will look like naked, and then believe it will happen. What you believe you can achieve.

34. Hang a piece of clothing such as a bikini or sexy outfit on a door handle or other visible place as reminder of what you will accomplish.

35. If your drive home from work takes you by your favorite fast-food restaurant or other eatery, find another route.

36. Eat a variety of foods in moderation; this will put a lid on your desire to overeat. Fill up on high-fiber foods too. They take up a lot of space in your stomach, so you're less likely to gorge on them.

37. Distract yourself with a non-food-related activity like exercising, reading, pursuing a favorite hobby, listening to music, writing letters, surfing the Internet (one of the best distractions yet), or soaking in a hot bath.

38. Make a list of 25 things to do other than eat. Keep your list handy.

39. Clear your kitchen cabinets of binge food.

40. Use nonstick saucepans for cooking so you don't have to add extra fat.

41. Eat your meals on smaller plates than usual; this will make it seem like you're eating more than you really are.

42. Keep plenty of cut-up crunchy raw vegetables around to snack on.

43. Freeze strawberries and other berries. They take longer to eat and provide a natural candy-like treat.

44. Never eat foods out of their original jars or containers; always eat them on a plate, sitting down at the dining table.

45. Tell your friends and family that you're on the Naked Fitness Nutrition Plan and that you need their support.

46. Grocery shop only from the list of foods allowed on the Naked Fitness Nutrition Plan.

47. Never go grocery shopping when you're hungry, but always on a full stomach. That way, you won't be tempted to buy something that would sabotage your diet.

48. Weigh yourself only once a week to keep from obsessing over your weight loss. Use the mirror to see how much body fat you're losing. It's much more motivating than the scale. But you can weight yourself daily as a tool to maintain your weight.

49. When you lose some pounds or achieve other important milestones while following the Naked Fitness Nutrition Plan, reward yourself with a nonfood treat or gift, something that makes you feel good about yourself and your appearance. Some ideas: a massage, a new pair of exercise shoes, new sports gear or equipment, a new exercise video, a weekend get-away, a shopping spree, a new outfit or bikini, a makeover at a day spa, a pedicure or manicure, a salon haircut, tickets to a concert, jewelry, a new CD or tape, a limousine ride to a concert or other event, an addition to something you collect, or an accessory or accent piece for your home. Treat yourself with things that don't cost money, like painting your nails, taking a walk to a friend's house, or even a bubble bath lit with candles.

50. Lose weight for yourself, not because your husband, mate, or parent wants you to.

10

THE NAKED FITNESS KEEP-IT-OFF PLAN

First, congratulations for following the workout and nutrition plan. You've made it through the program and you've reached your goals. I know you don't want to just be trim and look good naked. I know you want to stay trim and proud of your newly fit body.

Yet simple as this goal seems, it often eludes the most iron-willed of us. Sadly, most Americans are losing the battle of the bulge. Fifty-eight million people in the United States are 20 percent heavier than their ideal weight, and more than one-third are seriously overweight. The increases in obesity and disappointing rate of failure at weight control are not due to a lack of desire. Two million Americans spend approximately $10 million on weight loss programs annually—which proves we're motivated to lose weight—but only about 5 percent will keep the weight off for more than a year.

I'm always asking myself, Why are we doing such a poor job of solving the problem of obesity? We have the greatest number of choices of low-fat, nutritionally rich foods ever available. Home exercise equipment, video programs, and expert knowledge concerning diet and exercise are widely available. Yet not many buns (or any other body parts) of steel are evident in our population.

The formula for weight control is deceptively simple. Body weight equals energy in food intake minus energy expenditure (from maintenance of body processes, exercise, etc.).

Thus, a huge part of keeping your weight off has to do with what you eat from now on. I realize that when you finally reach your weight-loss goal, you can't wait to return to your old eating habits. But unless you've learned to make healthier food choices, returning to your old patterns usually results in regaining the lost weight. This can become an ongoing cycle of dieting to lose weight and then regaining it when the diet ends.

Transitioning from a weight-loss diet to an eating plan that maintains a healthy weight shouldn't require much of a change. If you lost weight on the Naked Fitness Nutrition Plan (and I know you did!), then adding a few foods back in should be all that's required to achieve weight maintenance. That's exactly what the Naked Fitness Keep-It-Off Plan does.

So let's step through each of the food groups and look at what—and how much—you can now add back in.

Fibrous Vegetables—Unlimited

Continue to stuff yourself with these! They're low in calories and high in fiber—plus loaded with health-enhancing benefits. Other foods you may now add in are these (please note serving sizes):

- Tomato juice – 1 cup
- Carrot juice – 1 cup
- Mixed vegetable juice – 1 cup
- Any freshly made vegetable juice – 1 cup

A note of caution: Don't overdo it. Restrict yourself to one cup a day of these juices.

Fruits—Two to Four Servings Daily

The Naked Fitness Keep-It-Off Plan liberalizes your fruit choices. Now you may include these foods (please note serving sizes):

100% Fruit Juices
Orange – ½ cup
Apple – ½ cup
Grape – ½ cup
Grapefruit – ½ cup

Other
Canned fruit (in water or its own juice) – ½ cup
Frozen fruit (unsweetened) – 1 cup

Light Proteins—Three Servings Daily

Continue to eat a serving of protein at each main meal to keep your metabolism running well. For weight control, it's best to continue to select proteins from the light proteins list because they are low in fat. However, feel free to add in lunch meats such as lean turkey, roast beef, ham, bologna, and salami as long as they are low-fat versions.

Try to enjoy some fish during the week. Remember, it's plentiful in omega-3 fats (as are green leafy vegetables, walnuts, walnut oil, canola oil, and flaxseed oil). If you're not crazy about fish, experts say fish oil capsules are an option. The most recent research raves about omega-3 fatty acids in the prevention of heart disease and stroke. In many cultures with high cold-water fish intakes, like that of the Inuit, heart disease and stroke are almost nonexistent.

Although there is no recommended daily allowance for omega-3, studies have shown that eating cold-water fish two to three times a week increases HDLs and decreases overall cholesterol levels.

Calcium-Rich Proteins—One to Two Servings Daily

Expand your choices to include the following:

Acidophilus milk – 1 cup
Buttermilk – 1 cup
Fat-free (skim) milk – 1 cup
Low-fat milk (1%) – 1 cup
Reduced-fat milk (2%) – 1 cup
Lactose-reduced milk – 1 cup
Lactose-free milk – 1 cup
Low-calorie or sugar-free puddings made with skim milk – ½ cup
Ice milk – ½ cup
Frozen yogurt – ½ cup
Ice cream, reduced-fat or reduced-sugar – ½ cup
Hard natural cheeses (cheddar, mozzarella, Swiss, parmesan, etc.) – 1 oz.
Ricotta cheese – ½ cup
Yogurt, fat-free – 1 cup
Yogurt, low-fat – 1 cup
Yogurt, reduced-fat – 1 cup
Yogurt, whole milk – 1 cup

Some additional tips:

- If you usually drink whole milk, switch gradually to fat-free milk to decrease saturated fat and calories. Try reduced-fat (2%), then low-fat (1%), and finally fat-free (skim).

- Add fat-free or low-fat milk instead of water to oatmeal and hot cereals.

- If you drink cappuccinos or lattes, ask for them with fat-free (skim) milk.

Starches—Zero to Three Servings Daily

Research suggests that for weight control, whole grains such as oats and brown rice have an advantage over highly processed, low-fiber grain products. Fiber-rich whole grains are more filling, and people who favor them over refined grains are more likely to have a normal body weight.

There are several reasons for this. Carbohydrates from foods such as whole grains contain various fibers and starches that may help regulate sugar levels in the bloodstream. These foods also may contain phytochemicals and enzyme inhibitors. All these factors can alter some metabolic reactions and decrease fat storage and may reduce the number of calories available to the body.

Avoid foods with white flour, even while on maintenance. They can raise your level of insulin, a hormone that signals your body to store carbohydrates as fat.

The Naked Fitness Keep-It-Off Plan expands your food choices to include these foods in the following serving sizes:

Grains, Cereals, and Pasta (Cooked or Ready to Eat)
Amaranth – ½ cup
Brown rice – ½ cup
Buckwheat – ½ cup
Bulgur (cracked wheat) – ½ cup
Cornmeal – ½ cup
Couscous – ½ cup
Enriched ready-to-eat cereal (Total, Special K, etc.) – 1 cup
Gluten-free bread – 1 slice
Gluten-free cereal – 1 cup
Gluten-free pasta – ½ cup
Granola, low-fat – ½ cup
Grits – ½ cup
High-fiber cereal (All Bran, Fiber One, etc.) – 1 cup
Millet – ½ cup
Oatmeal – ½ cup

Oat bran – ½ cup

Popcorn – 3 cups

Triticale – ½ cup

Whole-grain pita bread – 1 pocket

Whole-wheat or whole-grain bread – 1 slice

Whole-wheat crackers – 6 crackers

Whole-wheat pasta – ½ cup

Whole-wheat sandwich buns and rolls – 1 piece

Wild rice – ½ cup

Other Starches

Sweet potatoes – 1 medium

Yam – 1 medium

Beneficial Fats—One to Three Servings Daily

You may add the following fats:

Avocado – ¼ avocado

Butter – 1 tbsp.

Canola oil – 1 tbsp.

Corn oil – 1 tbsp.

Flaxseed oil – 1 tbsp.

Mayonnaise – 1 tbsp.

Mayonnaise, low fat – 2 tbsp.

Olive oil – 1 tbsp.

Peanut oil – 1 tbsp.

Safflower oil – 1 tbsp.

Sesame oil – 1 tbsp.

Soft tub or squeeze margarine with no trans fats* – 1 tbsp.

Sour cream – 1 tbsp.

Walnut oil – 1 tbsp.

---

* These man-made fats are found in margarine, shortening, and most packaged baked goods, crackers, and candies. The label tip-off is "hydrogenated" or "partially hydrogenated" appearing before any oil or fat. They are similar to saturated fats in their bad effects on the body.

To avoid regaining weight as you eat more beneficial fats, use them in place of heart-damaging saturated fats. To get you started:

- Skip the pepperoni (4 grams saturated fat per 3 oz.) and order your pizza topped with anchovies (1 gram omega-3 per 3 oz.) or veggies.

- Pick surf over turf: Instead of sirloin steak (6.4 grams saturated fat per 3 oz.), try salmon (1.2 grams omega-3 per 3 oz.).

- Instead of using bottled blue cheese dressing (1.5 grams saturated fat per tbsp.), make your own with olive oil (10.3 grams mono-unsaturates per tbsp.) or walnut oil (1.5 grams omega-3 per tbsp.).

- Stop sautéing in corn oil (9.8 grams saturated fat per tbsp.). Use canola oil (9.1 grams monounsaturates per tbsp.) instead.

- It's not necessarily better to dip bread in olive oil, because you're likely to eat too much oil and calories. Use a little butter instead, and you'll save calories.

- Ditch the sour cream dip (1.6 grams saturated fat per tbsp.); instead, eat celery, carrots, cucumbers, and other cut-up raw veggies with yogurt.

Planning Your Keep-It-Off Meals

The Naked Fitness Keep-It-Off Plan follows the same blueprint as the nutrition plan. For maintenance meal planning, simply follow this blueprint and add your food choices and daily serving guidelines. As a reminder, the blueprint appears at the top of the next page.

To help you, here is a sample Keep-It-Off daily menu:

Breakfast
1 cup high-fiber cereal
1 cup low-fat milk
½ cup 100% orange juice
Liquid glucosamine supplement, 1 serving

THE NAKED FITNESS MEAL BLUEPRINT

BREAKFAST
1 serving fresh fruit
1 light protein or calcium-rich protein
Liquid glucosamine supplement, 1 serving

SNACK
1 to 2 fruits

LUNCH
1 protein serving (4 to 6 oz.)
Fibrous vegetables

DINNER
1 protein serving (6 to 8 oz.)
Fibrous vegetables

OTHER
Add in 0 to 3 starch servings to any part of the menu
Add in 1 to 3 servings of beneficial fats to any part of the menu
Add in 1 to 2 servings of calcium-rich protein to any part of the menu

Snacks
6 whole wheat crackers with 1 oz. cheddar cheese
1 fresh fruit

Lunch
Caesar chicken salad: 1 grilled chicken breast on a mound of romaine lettuce; 4 tbsp. light Caesar salad dressing
½ cup ice milk

Dinner
8 oz. sirloin steak
1 medium baked potato with 1 tbsp. sour cream and chives
Steamed veggies

Strategies of the Slim and Successful

Research has shown that people who successfully lose weight and keep it off use a number of similar strategies. The five most common are:

- Strategy #1: Eat less fat (with an average of about 25 to 30 percent of calories from fat). The Naked Fitness Nutrition Plan and the Naked Fitness Keep-It-Off Plan accomplish that for you. Just stick to the guidelines and you'll stay in great shape.

- Strategy #2: Use monitoring techniques like weighing yourself frequently and tracking food intake. Try to weigh yourself weekly from now on. Research suggests that frequent weighing helps you lose more weight and keep it off. Give yourself a limit—say, a five-pound weight gain ceiling—you will not surpass. If your weight begins to creep up to that ceiling, spring into action right away by getting back to your plan.

- Strategy #3: Don't skip breakfast. Eating breakfast helps prevent overeating during other times of the day. Plus, it jumpstarts your metabolism for the whole day.

- Strategy #4: Graze during the day. Many successful dieters say they keep weight off by eating about five meals a day. They reported that 20 to 30 percent of their nutrients came from fat, 20 to 30 percent from protein, and the rest from carbohydrates—the same approach I recommend. The calorie levels of their weight-maintenance diets were similar to those during their weight loss. Successful weight maintenance diets also tend to be high in fiber.

- Strategy #5: Stay active (60 minutes or more of aerobic activity per day). In a study of people in the National Weight Control Registry (a database of people who have lost weight and kept it off for years), people reported burning an average of 3,000 calories weekly in exercise. That is the equivalent of walking four miles a day, seven days a week. Most of the subjects engaged in exercise more vigorous than walking. Their most frequent exercise was jogging, running, and aerobic dancing.

"Gentle" exercising such as the Naked Fitness alignment exercises and yoga have fat-burning advantages too. They build muscle, which boosts your metabolism, while emphasizing breathing and meditation. These, in turn, help reduce stress and balance hormones like cortisol that can cause weight gain.

These are all great strategies to employ—strategies that will keep your naked body trim and fit forever. Now here are a few of my own.

Go Ahead and Feast

Surprise! Feasting won't sabotage your weight-loss goals. The French, Italians, and other Europeans feast once or twice a week without gaining weight. Europeans can get away with this indulgence because they eat small meals the rest of the week. If you stick to slimming habits most of the week, feel free to splurge on a sumptuous brunch, order dessert after a meal out, or throw a dinner party on the weekends.

There is no "bad" food if you enjoy it once in a while, even fast-food burgers. Moderation is the key to success. Just be careful about the quantities you eat.

You have to stay flexible if you want to control your weight. No one can be 100 percent perfect all the time. It's okay to break the rules slightly when you need to. Just don't go overboard.

Watch Serving Sizes

Read the labels on packaged foods to determine their calories, which is what you need to pay attention to in order to lose weight and keep it off. My rule of thumb is to look first at the calories per serving and then check the serving size. You might be surprised by what the manufacturer considers a serving: For some cereals, like Grape-Nuts or certain brands of granola, it's only a half cup (compared to a cup and a quarter for Rice Krispies, say).

Don't Drink Too Many Calories

No one knows exactly why, but our bodies don't sense calories from liquids well. That signal failure can add up to a lot of pounds. Data from the Harvard Nurses' Health Study II, which studied 51,603 women, show that those who over a four-year period increased their intake of sugar-sweetened soft drinks from one or fewer a week to one or more a day added 358 daily calories and put on an average of 10 pounds. Even drinks that sound innocuous—vitamin-enriched water or fruit-flavored iced tea—may be deceptively high in calories. Read labels and calculate servings.

Don't Cave in to Cravings Too Often

Whether it's chocolate or chips, ice cream, or whipped cream, the foods we crave have one thing in common according to a recent Tufts University study: They are calorie-dense. But in that study, the researchers also noted that while virtually everyone has cravings, the dieters in the group who successfully lost weight and kept it off gave in to their must-haves less often. And when they did indulge, they kept portions reasonable. My advice is to accept that cravings are normal and then deal with them. Sometimes you can give in, and sometimes you need to wait for the desire to pass.

Devise a Plan

Come up with a plan for keeping your weight off. The worksheet in Appendix G will help you. All you have to do is record your thoughts and answers to my questions regarding why you want to stay Naked-Fitness trim and how you'll respond to any changes in your weight.

Don't Keep Your Plan a Secret

Support is the key to dropping pounds and keeping them off. That's why support groups and online diet communities work so well. But be careful whom you turn to: Canadian researchers recently interviewed people trying to change their diets and found that some spouses actively hindered the dieters' efforts (by eating forbidden foods in front of them, for example). If that sounds like someone in your household, try an online buddy.

Now that you've come this far, keep your new habits and don't look back. Forget the way you used to eat and continue with your plan. Be flexible, drink a lot of water, include plenty of veggies, and avoid overindulging. Continue working out with the same frequency that helped you drop the weight.

Our next stop on the path to Naked Fitness is to look at the some of the key obstacles that can prevent us from being our best, healthiest selves. I'll show you how to remove these obstacles from your life. That said, it's time to strip.

PART 4

Time
to
Strip

11

STRIP AWAY:
TIME BARRIERS

Most people—and research backs this up—say a lack of time is their biggest barrier to exercising and getting in shape. "There just aren't enough hours in the day" and "Who has the time?" are just a couple of responses that people give me when I ask them about their daily exercise routines.

People who say they don't have time to exercise aren't making it a priority. But if they realize what an impact exercise can have on their health, they may decide to make it a priority.

If you value your health, devote some time to exercise and move it up your priority list. The very first step to a healthier lifestyle is to stop making excuses about why you have no time to exercise. Procrastination gets you nowhere and keeps you overweight.

Finding the time to exercise doesn't have to be complicated. Any time can be the right time. The trick is to find a clever way to work an exercise routine into your everyday activities. Think about the minutes that turn into hours of TV watching. What about the time you spend surfing the Internet? You can use that time for exercising.

In the same way that we prioritize brushing our teeth, wearing clean underwear, and shaving, we can find time to make exercise a priority. In this chapter, I'll show you how.

To Choose Time Is to Save Time

Maybe you've bought into the myth that time controls us, when in reality we are in control. How we use that time is our choice, and we are free to make new choices any time. This doesn't mean there aren't consequences related to our decisions. When filling our time, then, our responsibility is to define our priorities, weigh the consequences, and make good choices.

It's not that we don't have time to exercise; the problem is that we need to better use the time we have. There are 168 hours in a week. You have the same 168 hours that I have. Shouldn't we be able to squeeze in at least three percent of those hours for exercise?

Absolutely. Take out your calendar, PDA, journal, a plain piece of paper, or the Charting My Day log in Appendix H. Start mapping one whole day ahead. Write in all your key activities, including appointments, volunteer activities, work hours, kids' activities, and so forth. Write down how you spend your time. How do you normally spend weekends? Sleeping in? Watching television? Visiting with friends? How much television do you watch? What sedentary activities do you engage in?

Next, circle the important activities that you must do each day, meaning you couldn't function if you did not complete these tasks. Then red-line the activities you feel are time wasters—activities or tasks you could eliminate or delegate. These represent minutes you can free up for health and exercise priorities.

Look at your current schedule and determine how you can rearrange it to accommodate an exercise routine. As you do, you'll begin to see where your time goes each week and how you might often spend time doing nothing. You'll see all the free time you really have. It's merely hiding in your day! I think you'll be surprised to discover that there's plenty of time for exercise.

You always have enough time if you use it wisely. Your dilemma goes deeper than having a shortage of time; remember, it's basically an issue of priorities. Most people leave undone those things that should be done, while they do things that they shouldn't be doing. You can take back your day.

How I Reclaimed My Schedule

People always ask me, "How do you find the time?" I say, "I make the time." Here are a few things I have done to free up time in my schedule:

- I eliminate email clutter by opting out of as many ads, newsletters, and message groups as I can. I seek out information only if I really want to know about something. This is kind of like shopping for what you need instead of browsing and impulse buying.

- I replaced my formal bedding setup with a comforter and two pillows, so I spend less time in the morning making my bed. The comforter is so warm, it doesn't need any extra sheets or blankets, which saves me at least 10 minutes making my bed each morning and lightens my laundry load. Plus, this time-saving switch makes my bedroom look fresher and neater, and I feel better coming home to my neatly made bed every night.

- I set alarms for when I need to stop doing any activity that can really wait until tomorrow. That's how I deal with projects that need a little time each day to tackle so I don't wait until the last minute. Sometimes I would get lost trying to accomplish one task in a single day just so I could get it off my list. Setting that timer helped me move on to other tasks and actually get the jobs done faster.

- I replaced the towel bars in my bathroom with hooks. This arrangement still looks neat, and it takes me less time to hang up and drape my towels.

- I've trained my kids to be responsible for themselves, once they can read or reach the kitchen counter, no matter how young they are. I've taught them how to prepare cereal, toast bread and frozen waffles, and use the microwave oven. I've shown my children how to do their own laundry. My kids are so incredibly talented on a computer, why not take on the washer and dryer? They also have chores around the

SHOP-ILATES™: TIME-SAVING EXERCISES ON THE GO

STEP 1—POSTURE PUSH

This key Shop-ilates™ move is perfect for the grocery store. Start with your hands shoulder-width apart on your shopping cart, and use your lats, shoulders, and hands together to work on your chest and shoulders.

While you wait in line or throughout your shopping trip, try for 20 repetitions of pushing and pulling your cart (add a small child or 25-pound turkey for resistance) while standing in place. Exhale on the push and inhale on the pull.

STEP 2—PARKED PERFECT

Stuck in traffic? While in a parked position, use your headrest to help strengthen the back of your neck. Pull your chin down and lift tall through the top of your head as you press back gently against the head-rest. As a passenger, you can practice this simple neck strengthening exercise for 10- to 30-second holds as you travel. You'll experience less pressure on your mid and lower back and, as a positive side effect, better posture.

house like taking out the garbage, picking out and organizing dinner, clearing dishes, mowing the lawn, and doing other tasks that help everyone in the family. If you don't have children, ask your partner, spouse, or roommate to help around the house. That way, everyone in the household has more time.

- I leave dishes in the sink until the evening. In other words, I do only one kitchen clean-up, and that's at night so that I'll wake up to a neat kitchen the next morning. A tidy kitchen sets the tone for my entire day. I know some of you may not be able to let this one go, but I have learned that it's perfectly okay to leave dishes alone during the day. They don't invite bugs into the house or cause any other issues. I don't,

SHOP-ILATES™: TIME-SAVING EXERCISES ON THE GO (continued)

STEP 3—SHOULDER MATTERS

Even a "small" wheeled suitcase can weight up to 50 pounds. Think twice about how you move, because your shoulders matter. Gripping the extended handle of your "wheelie bag" or small cart with your palm facing forward while you pull it behind you can injure or tear rotator cuff muscles. Instead, push your luggage or bend your arm as you pull it along with the palm facing backward, thumb toward the body. Using the luggage like a washboard (forward and back pushes to the front or behind you) can tone up those triceps and prevent "Bingo Betty" arms. Try for 20 repetitions both front and back on each arm.

STEP 4—BAG IT

Use those filled-up shopping bags as muscle toners. Start with your arms bent at the elbow, resting on your hips with bags in hand. Slowly reach your hands forward with palms upward. Alternate forward reaches for 20 repetitions. This will strengthen your shoulders and biceps and help with your upper back posture.

---

however, leave dishes or messes in the house for days on end. A bad housekeeping habit like that would end up costing me time in the long run.

- I do a load of laundry every day to stay on top of my chores. And I let my ironing pile up for at least two months before I get to it, unless it's an emergency need-to-wear-it outfit. Fortunately, I have very little ironing because I buy wrinkle-free clothes.

- I always keep at least one workout outfit, socks, and training shoes in my car—and deodorant and perfume too—just in case I can't get to a place with a shower. I can still get in a stretch or walk without being too sweaty and feel like I did something for myself.

- I exercise on the go, even while shopping (see the section on my Shop-ilates™ routine on pages 204–205). I might do a wall squat in the elevator or walk fast up an escalator or tighten my tummy muscles while standing in line. Every little bit helps.

- I say "yes" to not cooking. I triple my recipes, for example, and freeze dinners. My favorites are my tortilla soup and polenta chili (recipes are in Appendix F). Both take less than 30 minutes to make, and I do them at the same time. Cook enough for two or three dinners and then freeze and defrost as needed. This way, most energy-intensive cooking is done once for several meals. As for frozen microwave veggies, they're a staple in my household.

- I am a master multitasker. I always double up on duties: I unload the dishwasher while I talk on the phone, vacuum the rugs while the washing machine is running, and soak pans in soapy water while dinner is cooking.

More Ways to Strip Away Time Barriers

If you feel like your leisure time has shrunk, leaving less time to exercise, here are several more tips to help you beat the clock.

START EARLY

Get up an hour or half-hour earlier than normal and start exercising. (Have at least a piece of fruit first for energy.) By working out early in the morning, you get your exercise session over with, and that feels empowering. Plus, exercise will energize you mentally and physically for the rest of the day. Try going to the gym at 6 a.m., for example, while everyone else is still asleep. Return home before your spouse leaves for work, allowing plenty of time to feed your family breakfast.

SQUEEZE IN SHORTER WORKOUTS

Try exercising in 10-minute bouts throughout the day. Researchers at Stanford University divided men into two groups: One group ran three times a day for 10 minutes, and the other ran 30 minutes once a day. After eight weeks, the two groups had comparable fitness gains in endurance and weight loss. Many other studies show that 10-minute bouts of activity can produce highly beneficial metabolic changes and can produce healthy rewards comparable to those achieved with much more rigorous exercise regimens, such as lowered cholesterol and reduced blood pressure. Shorter workouts can do as much good as longer exercise sessions, and they're definitely better than doing no exercise at all.

EXERCISE IN DISGUISE

You can always find ways to incorporate physical activity into your day. For example, take the stairs whenever you can, walk your dog, or put on your favorite music and dance. Pop in an exercise video while your toddler naps or before your spouse wakes up. Do you like to watch television during the day? Walk around the house or up and down your stairs every time a commercial comes on. Doing yard work, washing your car, or painting your walls will burn calories, too, as long as you do them regularly.

Don't forget to use your pedometer to keep track of how many steps you take in a day. Work in more steps by walking around in the airport instead of sitting while waiting for a plane, for example, or by strolling the field while you watch your kids play soccer.

Physical activity doesn't always have to be scheduled or expensive. Simple changes in behavior, such as taking the stairs once or twice a day, go a long way toward physical fitness.

BURN CALORIES ON THE ROAD

Keeping a commitment to exercise while you're on the road is not always easy. But travel is no excuse to go to flab. Some suggestions:

- Find a hotel with a fitness center. Hotel fitness centers are spreading like, well, an untended midriff. Thousands of American hotels now have fitness facilities where you can get in aerobic and resistance training workouts. If the hotel doesn't have a gym, find out if it is affiliated with one nearby and exercise there.

TIME-SAVING SIT-ILATES™

The typical office worker is in his or her chair approximately six hours a day, and according to a study published in *Current Cardiovascular Risk Results*, prolonged sitting is a "distinct health hazard." To combat the ill health effects of "sitting a lot at ease," improve your alignment, and squeeze in some exercise time, I have created Sit-ilates™, pronounced sit-i-lot-ees.

These simple exercises based on Joseph Pilates' principles of spine alignment, breath, and body posture are a great way to improve your physique with very little time. Sit-ilates™ helps stretch and strengthen your muscles to help prevent arthritis and lower back pain and improve your posture. I have organized these movements from top to bottom, and you can do them right in your office or at home.

STEP 1—CHEST STRETCH

Sit tall with your feet on the ground. Grasp your hands at the back of your chair and widen across the chest as you squeeze your shoulder blades together. Inhale as you raise your rib cage away from your hips and then curl your chin down to your chest and exhale, contracting your abdominals and widening through your back. Repeat 10 times.

STEP 2—SPINE ROTATION

Sit tall with your feet on the ground. Lift any 5- to 10-pound object (e.g., gallon of milk, a laptop, or small weight) with arms extended out in front of you. Lift the rib cage and inhale. Exhale as you rotate the object to

- If you want to strike out on both fronts, take to the streets safely and wisely. Try to find a safe place where you can walk or jog. When you get back to your room, do three sets each of push-ups, three sets of abdominal crunches, and three sets of squats and lunges. You'll have pretty much done a total body workout without any equipment.

TIME-SAVING SIT-ILATES™ (continued)

your right. Keep your shoulders relaxed and inhale as you return to center. Repeat on the other side and perform 10 reps.

STEP 3—SEATED V BALANCE

Sit at the edge of your chair and lean slightly back off your sit bones. Staying tall and wide through your chest, inhale as you draw your knees up; exhale as you extend your legs, keeping them just a few inches off the floor for beginners and higher for the more advanced. Repeat 10 times.

STEP 4—REVERSE PLANK

Place your hands on the side of your chair's seat and walk your legs out forward with hips on the chair. Inhale to prepare and then exhale as you lift your hips up, squeezing the backs of your thighs and hips. Hold for one to two seconds and return to a seated position as you inhale. Repeat 10 times. This exercise should be done on a stationary chair.

STEP 5—SEATED ROLL UP

Sit tall with your feet on the ground and shoulder-width apart, arms extended in front of you. Inhale as your curl your chin to your chest and slowly roll down between your knees to the floor. Reaching out and forward, exhale as you roll your spine one vertebrae at a time up to seated position. Lift your body slowly, feeling yourself lifting and stacking each vertebrae separately. Repeat 10 times.

• You can easily pack portable fitness equipment such as resistance tubing. Tubing reproduces the workout you'd get from free weights or machines at a gym; they provide the resistance you need to effectively work most of your muscle groups. Tubing exercises help target specific body parts.

- Toting your laptop on your trip? Don't forget to pack some exercise DVDs. You'll have your own exercise classes with you. DVDs are an excellent in-room workout option.

I travel frequently for business, and I always schedule exercise into my travel itineraries. Here's how I managed to fit in exercise recently while away on business in Colorado:

5:15 a.m.: Wake up.

6 a.m.: Teach a poolside class on how to manage and treat your back pain.

7:30 a.m.: Enjoy a nonfat latte at the coffee shop.

8:30 a.m.: Have a carton of yogurt.

10 a.m.: Arrive at a conference for school administrators. For exercise I walked the corridors of the conference center for 30 minutes.

10:30 a.m: Teach the conference.

11:30 a.m.: Drive to Colorado Springs to meet my sister, niece, and nephew for lunch and shopping.

1 p.m.: Shopping at the mall. (Mall shopping counts as exercise! I walked as briskly as I could from store to store.)

4 p.m.: Head to the airport.

11:30 p.m.: Arrive home in Chicago.

For most of us, no day is typical. But with some creative planning, there's always a way to be more active and make it count.

SCHEDULE YOUR EXERCISE APPOINTMENT

Write on your calendar or planner the days and times you will formally exercise, such as going to the gym or attending an exercise class. In other words, schedule your workouts as you would any other appointment. This will help you devote time and establish a regular routine. And, if possible, try to exercise the same time each day, because research shows that people are more likely to exercise routinely if they stick to a set time. Set aside at least 30 minutes each day just for you. Use that time to exercise. Treating exercise like an appointment will help you stick to your regimen.

WORK OUT AT THE OFFICE

All across America, companies are setting up wellness programs for their employees, and many of these programs offer exercise facilities and classes. If your company has an on-site exercise program, take advantage of it— before work, during your lunch hour, or after work.

The American work week gets longer each year. More time in the office means less time to exercise, more time sitting, and probably more stress. At your desk or in your office, you can still squeeze in some exercises when you're crunched for time. These include 30 seconds to one minute of cardiovascular exercise such as jumping jacks or step-ups using stairs, a bench, or a chair. If you have time for lunch, you have time to exercise. Or try my Sit-ilates™ workout, described in the box on pages 208–209.

GET HELP

Friends and family are an important source of support as you pursue a healthier lifestyle. See whether your spouse or another family member is willing to help you with a household task or child care while you exercise. Or join a gym that offers babysitting. If it's affordable, hire a housekeeper to save time. Or barter for a better body. Offer to walk your neighbor's dog in exchange for babysitting so that you have even more time to work out.

By identifying available time and stripping away time barriers, you'll feel much better about committing to a more active lifestyle. We all have time to exercise. We really do. So don't serve time; make time serve you.

12

STRIP AWAY:
TOXIC LIFESTYLE HABITS

Maybe you've wrestled with the same 15 or 30 pounds or more for years—weighed and measured foods like a chemist, tried everything from low-fat to high-protein. And here you are again, struggling to zip up your favorite pair of jeans. You know it's time to get serious about slimming down, but at this point you just feel stuck. It's not nearly as hard as you might think. The key is to strip away certain toxic lifestyle and dietary habits that have stood in your way to lasting weight loss and a body that looks fabulous in the buff. Here goes.

Toxic Lifestyle Habit #1: Sleep Deprivation

How long and how well you sleep affects hormones that regulate your appetite and body weight. A large, ongoing research effort called the Wisconsin Sleep Cohort Study found that people who sleep less weigh more. Sleeping only four to five hours a night—instead of the recommended seven to eight—alters levels of the appetite-regulating hormones leptin and ghrelin, leading to increased appetite.

Leptin is a key element in the body's weight-regulation system. When your system works properly, leptin and other chemicals trigger the area in your brain that lets you know you're full. But when the system malfunctions and your brain blocks messages from these hormones, you won't feel full even when you have consumed an adequate amount of food. Ghrelin is called the "hunger hormone" because it makes us hungry. Levels reliably spike as mealtimes approach.

Also, when you're sleep-deprived, your body produces higher levels of a stress hormone called cortisol. Similar to adrenaline, it keeps you alert and clearheaded but causes sugar and caffeine cravings. Cortisol also appears to trigger fat storage around your tummy.

Sleeping plays a major role in your overall health. It gives your body a chance rejuvenate and renew itself. During sleep, your body can heal injuries and infections, eliminate toxins and waste products, dissipate stress, and replenish fuel stores in your muscle fibers and bloodstream. Sleep also allows your immune system to recharge so that you're better protected from disease. What's more, sleep revives you mentally. It improves your productivity and creativity and restores your brain functions, including information processing. Sleep is an absolute requirement for good health and a great-looking naked body.

If you're extremely overweight, the added pounds will definitely interfere with your sleep. Imagine placing a 20-pound weight on your chest and then trying to get a good night's rest. Being overweight or obese is associated with sleep apnea, which is interrupted breathing during sleep. When apnea occurs, not enough air reaches the lungs. This causes the heart to work harder, blood pressure to increase, and abnormalities in sugar metabolism to emerge. Fortunately, sleep apnea can be cured by weight loss and treated with a breathing apparatus.

So to get fit and stay fit, you must get sound shut-eye. If you're having trouble achieving that kind of slumber, here are some practical tips:

- Make it a habit to get to bed around 9:00 to 10:00 p.m., when your body naturally secretes the hormone melatonin. Melatonin, which is also available as a dietary supplement, helps regulate leptin levels. As noted above, leptin is an appetite-regulating hormone.

TO NAP OR NOT TO NAP?

If you are sleep-deprived, taking a nap is a good idea. In fact, it may help you shed pounds and stay healthy. A Harvard study published in the *Archives of Internal Medicine* revealed that people who regularly napped at least three times a week for an average of 30 minutes had a 37 percent lower risk of heart attack than those who didn't nap. Napping also contributes to weight loss according to a study in the *American Journal of Physiology, Endocrinology, and Metabolism*. That study looked at hormone levels in 41 men and women who were part of a seven-day sleep-deprivation experiment. Those allowed to nap for two hours following a night without any sleep showed a significant drop in cortisol, a hormone related to high levels of stress, and a complement of growth hormone, which helps regulate insulin and fat storage. Researchers concluded that a mid-afternoon nap improves alertness and performance and reverses the negative metabolic effects of sleep loss.

- Try not to exercise two to three hours prior to bedtime. While exercise makes you more alert, it also causes your body temperature to rise, so finish your exercising at least three hours before bedtime. Late afternoon workouts are best for a restful night's sleep.
- Enjoy some warm milk. Scientists don't know why exactly, but drinking warm milk or warm decaffeinated tea before going to bed helps set your body up for sleep. Some research suggests that the amino acid tryptophan in milk may have a role in helping you sleep. Tryptophan is involved in increasing levels of the brain chemical serotonin, which is a calming chemical.
- Coordinate your sleep with light and darkness. Try to sleep when the sun goes down or darken your room. Allowing too much light in your room while you're trying to sleep interferes with the production of melatonin.
- Eliminate electromagnetic fields (like cell phone chargers, lights, TV's, and other electrical devices) from your nightstand and sleep area. Electronic gizmos emit bright light into your bedroom. Even digital

clocks can put out more light than you need. All that light disturbs the normal rhythm of the hormones preparing your body for sleep.

- Declutter your bedroom. We spend one-third of our lives sleeping, so our bedrooms should be peaceful retreats. By paying attention to the neatness of your room, you'll be on your way to a better night's sleep.

- Keep your room cool. About four hours after you drift off to sleep, your body temperature drops to its lowest level, and your room should match what's going on in your system. The ideal sleep temperature falls between 60 to 65 degrees Fahrenheit. Most people say they sleep better in the winter, which makes sense because a cool bedroom contributes to better sleep.

- Sleep naked! Your birthday suit is the perfect temperature regulator compared to cotton, Lycra, satin, and other pajama material.

- Come up with a personal bedtime ritual just like you would for your children. Take a warm bath, listen to soft music, read, meditate, or do something spiritual before turning out the lights.

- Set a regular bedtime so your biological clock gets used to a routine sleep pattern.

- Avoid or cut down on caffeine, alcohol, and tobacco; all disrupt sleeping patterns, making it difficult to drift off or stay asleep. Eating too much food close to bedtime affects many people's slumber as well.

- Plan your next day's schedule before going to bed. Also, count your blessings (rather than sheep); this calms your mind. Avoid anxiety-provoking activities like working, paying bills, or having serious talks right before bedtime.

- Count backward from 300 by 3s with a deep breath between each number.

- Listen to white noise generated by the steady, low whir of a fan or a noise machine. It can help drown out any disruptive clamor.

- Try natural sleep aids such as melatonin or valerian. Check with your doctor for your best options.

- Relax and get fit at the same time by performing my Sleep-ilates™ moves, explained on the facing page.

SLEEP-ILATES™ FOR A GREAT NIGHT'S SLEEP

If you have trouble falling asleep, try these exercises to put your body in alignment so you can get a little more shut-eye. Restorative exercises like these trigger the parasympathetic nervous system to activate the relaxation response. Do them before nodding off to bed.

BUTTERFLY

Take two large towels, fold them in half, and then roll them into cylinders. Lie on the ground with one towel between your shoulder blades and supporting your heart and the other towel just below your belt line.

Bring the bottom of your feet together with knees to the sides and arms open. Take 10 deep breaths and relax the body.

CROSSOVER

Start by lying on the floor or a firm surface with your legs extended and arms open to the side. Bend one knee up toward the hips and cross it over your body.

Breathe deeply as you straighten your leg, keeping it crossed over your body. Inhale as you bend the knee back to center and exhale as you straighten your leg to the floor.

Alternate sides for a series of 10 repetitions.

SPINE ROLL

Start in a seated position with your knees tucked in to your chest. Slowly roll back until your shoulder blades touch the ground and then roll back up.

Repeat 10 times.

Toxic Lifestyle Habit #2: Irregular Meal Patterns

Eating regular meals each day boosts your health, keeps your weight under control, and energizes your body. When the body is fed at regular intervals, the brain sends signals that calories don't have to be packed away as fat. Skipping meals, on the other hand, sends a signal to the body that there's a famine underway and calories should be hoarded as a defense against starvation.

How many meals should you eat each day? Three large meals or multiple small meals? Despite more than 40 years of research into the question of whether eating three large meals or multiple small meals is best, no clear consensus has emerged. That's because something much more basic is at work: calories. Whether you eat three meals or five or six, weight loss ultimately comes down to how much energy is consumed, not how often or how regularly you eat. So it's perfectly okay to enjoy three squares a day or nosh on multiple mini-meals. One of the biggest concerns I have about mini-meals is that the more meals you allow in your day, the more opportunity you have to overeat. So be careful.

I can't say this enough: Among meals, breakfast is the most important. Numerous studies point to the importance of breaking the overnight fast with food. And no, breakfast doesn't have to be eaten immediately upon rising, although there's evidence to suggest that consuming food within an hour or so of waking helps keep blood sugar levels even and insulin production steady and reduces hunger. Members of the National Weight Control Registry, a group of more than 5,000 people who have successfully lost at least 30 pounds and kept it off for at least three years, report that eating breakfast is key to their efforts.

Skipping breakfast is more toxic than you might realize. Research has shown that this bad habit results in greater consumption of calories, higher levels of total blood cholesterol and low-density lipoprotein—one of the most dangerous types of cholesterol—and changes in insulin sensitivity that can lead to weight gain.

The best breakfast, one that's high in lean protein such as eggs or yogurt, helps many people feel full and eat less throughout the day. Eating carbohydrates such as muffins, bagels, or toast is more likely to boost your appetite later in the day.

Toxic Lifestyle Habit #3: Food Cravings

Among the toughest obstacles to weight loss are hunger and cravings. But even these are easier to beat than you might think. It all comes down to food selection. Processed carbs, including most cereals, pastas, and breads, not to mention sugar-laden desserts, create their own cravings by elevating insulin in the body. Insulin is the hormone that allows the muscles to convert sugar into energy. If the body receives too much sugar, the pancreas will produce more insulin to compensate for the extra sugar levels. But wildly oscillating levels of sugar and insulin lead to further sugar cravings, which starts the whole process again. High blood sugar and high levels of insulin put you on what I like to call the craving express. It's a blood sugar roller-coaster ride that never ends well. Over time, the pancreas will work harder to produce enough insulin to combat all the sugar, and type 2 diabetes can result.

One of the best ways to keep your food urges under control is to mix up your meals. This means having a few ounces of lean protein with a serving of complex carbohydrates and a bit of healthy fat. This mixture helps keep blood sugar and insulin levels steady. The Naked Fitness Nutrition Plan helps keep all these factors in check.

Complex carbohydrates such as whole grains, legumes, vegetables, and fruit are packed with fiber, which also helps regulate blood sugar. Fiber makes you feel full, so you're less likely to stuff yourself on high-calorie foods. What's more, the fiber found in foods such as bran, whole-wheat products, and oats naturally binds to the fats you eat and helps escort them from the body. The net effect is a reduction in the number of calories left behind that can be stored as body fat.

Protein also elicits its own hormonal response by elevating levels of the hormone glucagon. Glucagon opposes the action of insulin and actually unlocks fat stores. To me, glucagon, means glucose (sugar), be gone! It allows the body to utilize the sugar instead of having it hang out in the bloodstream.

Even if you are vegan, you need protein. Nuts, beans, and legumes are great protein sources. You can still eat enough protein by combining many different vegetables and grains. A few smart choices: banana with yogurt, soup with beans and a whole-grain cracker, low-fat or nonfat yogurt with fruit.

Identify the times of day when you start to reach for fattening foods, and then preempt the problem by scheduling a healthy snack a half-hour earlier. It may sound counterintuitive, but eating an apple or a low-fat yogurt right before heading out to a restaurant will help you avoid overeating once you're there, since you won't be starving when you arrive.

Think before you eat and consider your choices. Just by switching from a "want or crave" response, you will turn on different neurotransmitters in your brain to help you stay on track.

Toxic Lifestyle Habit #4: Portion Distortion

We eat too much and we wonder why we have a weight problem. Portion size is vital to weight control, because the bigger the meal, the more calories you consume. And remember that if you don't burn off all the calories you eat, no matter how healthy they are, you will gain weight or find it nearly impossible to lose weight.

The upward trend in portion sizes has finally been recognized for its part in super-sizing our waistlines. Government studies tell us that the average number of calories Americans eat each day has risen from 1,854 to 2,002 during the past 20 years. That increase of 148 calories per day works out to 15 pounds of extra weight each year.

These days, dinner plates and bowls are unnecessarily large, making it difficult to tell if you've just dished up one serving of pasta or four. Restaurants serve mountains of food, and in many cases the servers bring bottomless baskets of bread to the table before the meal even begins. The food industry has increased the standard serving sizes for items like juice and soda from 12 ounces 20 years ago to 20- and even 24-ounce bottles today. Servings were even smaller in the fifties and sixties. The competitive fast-food industry offers more food for fewer dollars in a bid to win customers. It's good for their business but not so good for your waistline.

People tend to eat what's put on their plate, even if they know it's larger than a typical portion. At least one study published in the *American Journal of Clinical Nutrition* showed that when a group of people was given smaller portions, that's all they ate. When they were given bigger portions, they cleaned their plates, without feeling any fuller than when they ate smaller portions.

When you eat out, order smart: lean meat, vegetables, and a whole-grain side. Or put half of your meal into a take-out container and close the lid before you take your first bite. Also, order regular or small portions, not the super-duper, mega-sized options. Ask your waiter about the size of the appetizers and entrees. If the portions tend to be large, split an entrée with a friend or order an appetizer as your main course.

When dining at home, try switching to slightly smaller dinnerware or purchase portion-control dinnerware, which is available from several companies. Three ounces of pasta on a 10-inch plate looks like a good amount, but on a 12-inch plate it looks like an appetizer.

Change your perceptions of portion sizes by using visual comparisons such as:

- Three ounces of meat, poultry, or fish is about the size of the palm of a woman's hand or the size of a deck of cards.

- Half a cup of rice, pasta, vegetables, or cut fruit is about the size of a small fist.

- An ounce of cheese is about the size of a typical thumb.

- One cup of chopped fresh greens is about the size of a small hand holding a tennis ball.

At the supermarket, read package labels, which indicate how much of the product equals one serving. Some smaller packages, like snack-size bags of chips, may look like a single serving but actually contain a lot more.

Ultimately, you should determine the right portion size by how full you are and not by the amount of food in front of you. That will allow you to push back from the table when you feel satisfied instead of when your plate is clean.

Toxic Lifestyle Habit #5: Environmental Vulnerability

Being overweight and out of shape is an environmental issue. We live in a world that promotes eating huge quantities of food while doing less and less all the time. It is not easy to make good food choices in certain surroundings. For every step forward you take, your food environment can send you back two steps. But it doesn't have to! Your home environment—where you store food, cook food, and eat food—is the environment over which you have the most control. If you can take charge of your home, this action alone can take you most of the way toward losing weight and keeping it off. Yes, this is tough, because most people are very attached to the way they live. But when you get a handle on the immediate world around you, you won't be vulnerable to those things that make you gain weight. When you can eliminate or at least control certain situations—and you can—then you can prevent the behavior that typically follows (like overeating or not exercising). In other words, you can redesign your environment so that it supports healthy choices. Here are some strategies to help you:

- Clear out high-calorie, tempting binge foods from your pantry or refrigerator—everything that threatens to wreck your resolve, including ice cream, left-over pie, and pizza. If it's there, you'll be tempted to eat it, so toss it or hide it in a container. If you don't see it, it's much easier to avoid.

- Don't go grocery shopping when you're hungry, and avoid the snack-food aisles to steer clear of temptations.

- Buy only healthy foods and stick to your Naked Fitness shopping lists. If you must buy fattening foods for the nondieters in your family, purchase versions you don't care for. For example, if you like chocolate chip cookies, buy another type of cookie for your family that will be easy for you to pass up.

- Have healthy snacks like yogurt, a small serving of nuts, or a piece of fresh fruit on hand so you're never famished.

- Choose a route to and from work that doesn't involve passing your favorite fast-food restaurant, ice cream parlor, bakery, or other place that has caused trouble in the past. Avoiding situations that prompt overeating can go a long way toward helping you lose weight.

- Stock your kitchen with appliances designed for healthy cooking, for example, a vegetable steamer or an indoor grill. When you have ready access to the tools and appliances that make your life easier and your eating more nutritious, you'll use them.

- Find ways to minimize the time you spend in the kitchen.

- Discard leftovers or pass them along to coworkers.

- Designate certain areas in your home as "eating only" zones, such as the kitchen and dining-room tables, and don't eat anywhere else in your house. Many people I've worked with who are successful at losing and keeping off weight have only one or two places in their home that are designated for eating. They don't eat anywhere else—not in front of the TV, not standing in front of the refrigerator, not in bed, not in the car.

- Take up a hobby like knitting or needlepoint that you can do while watching TV if that's when you are in the habit of nibbling.

- Make social plans so you're not home by yourself and tempted to overeat.

As you look over these five toxic habits, take an honest inventory of any that are blocking your way. From there, formulate a plan to strip them away so you can attain your Naked Fitness goals.

13

STRIP AWAY: STRESS

I love to tell the story of the lecturer who was explaining stress management to an audience. He raised a glass of water and asked, "How heavy is this glass of water?"

Hands went up, and people guessed at weight. Answers ranged from 4 ounces to 20 ounces.

The lecturer replied, "The absolute weight doesn't matter. It depends on how long you try to hold it."

The room was silent as he continued his explanation.

"If I hold it for a minute, that's not a problem.

"If I hold it for an hour, I'll have an ache in my right arm.

"If I hold it for a day, you'll have to call an ambulance. In each case, it's the same weight, but the longer I hold it, the heavier it becomes."

He went on, "And that's the way it is with stress management. If we carry our burdens all the time, sooner or later, as the burden becomes increasingly heavy, we won't be able to carry on. As with the glass of water, you have to put it down for a while and rest before holding it again. When we're refreshed, we can carry on with the burden. So, before you return home tonight, put the burden of work down. Don't carry it home. You can pick it up tomorrow.

"Whatever burdens you're carrying now, let them down for a moment if you can. Put down anything that may be a burden to you right now. Don't pick it up again until after you've rested a while."

Excellent advice, wouldn't you agree?

These days, we are carrying many stressors: economy, career, family, health, and the list goes on. Even trying to get in shape is stressful because we know that if we don't, we are putting ourselves at risk of developing many serious illnesses including heart disease, cancer, and diabetes.

Stress is something we live with daily—the result of the many demands and pressures in our lives. It's a normal reaction to upheaval, emotional upset, or simply too many demands on our time. Stress is good for your body when it motivates you to accomplish your goals. And it serves a defensive purpose in times of danger. When you suddenly find yourself in a threatening situation the stress of that moment incites your body to kick into high gear and do something. This is called the "fight or flight response," and it's triggered by the autonomic nervous system. Your brain releases the stress hormones, cortisol and adrenaline, into your system. As a result, your heart beats faster, blood pressure rises, muscles tense, your senses become more acute, and blood sugar is mobilized for energy. Your entire body has made all the metabolic preparations necessary to respond to an attack. However, all too often, the attack you are responding to is a major stressor such as job loss, a birth or a death, or a divorce or a minor stressor such as bouncing a check or being stuck in traffic.

This response gets us over life's hurdles every day, but problems arise when stress is chronic and unresolved and your body stays primed to react. This can wreak havoc with your physical well-being. Stress suppresses the immune system and is a contributing factor in many diseases including heart disease, kidney disease, gastrointestinal disorders, back pain, headaches, insomnia, and depression.

Stress can not only cause serious illnesses. Did you know it can also cause your body to lay down more flab, especially around your middle?

This occurs for several reasons. Stress can cause depression, and this type of depression is associated with elevated levels of cortisol and weight gain. In the body, chronic stress kicks cortisol production into high gear. The stress-induced release of cortisol activates certain fat-storing pathways and encourages your body to store more fat, particularly around the abdomen. If you're constantly under stress and your body is producing higher than normal levels of cortisol, you may become thicker around the middle.

Cortisol also triggers a hike in insulin levels, causing an increase in appetite-stimulating brain chemicals. At the same time, blood levels of serotonin drop. Serotonin is a general mood regulator that's manufactured in the brain from the amino acid tryptophan, along with some help from the B vitamins.

Stress-triggered depression is also associated with binging behaviors, which can definitely boost weight. Some people with depression are also less physically active, and this affects weight, too.

Studies show that most people hanker for more high-fat and sweet foods during times of worry, anxiety, and tension. These foods typically have more calories and contribute to weight gain.

And if stress affects your sleep, causing insomnia or unrefreshing sleep, this can promote the release of cortisol. Poor sleep can also affect other hormones such as ghrelin and leptin, which affect eating behaviors.

Charla, age 31, is one of my many clients who have stress-associated weight issues. Her biggest problem, and the reason she ballooned to 187 pounds, was stress eating. Her life was endlessly crazy: working two jobs, raising a small child as a single mom, and just trying to keep it all together. As she told me, "All I want to do at night is slump on the couch and eat pizza and ice cream!" Her overeating was fueled by emotions, and she had trouble making good choices.

Embarrassed by her growing size, Charla started to withdraw from social situations. "I was uncomfortable going out with friends and meeting guys," she said. She reached her personal rock bottom when she woke up one Saturday unable to fit into yet another pair of pants. "I sobbed for hours."

After her breakdown, Charla did some much needed soul-searching. "I told myself, 'This is enough,'" she said. "I couldn't keep living like this. I had to make a change."

It was a heartbreaking, challenging time for Charla, but I reassured her that she could stop stress eating with a few well-chosen strategies. I suggested that she first concentrate on stripping away her stress.

Using many of the suggestions I offer below, Charla learned to deal with certain stressors before she reached mental overload (and plate overload). Fitting in her two hours of walking every day was a great fix, and she found that during moments of frenzy, simply taking time to sit quietly and breathe deeply for a few minutes helped diffuse her tension.

She lost 60 pounds in five months. Since shedding the pounds, she's learned to find balance in her life, and she's even found a way to deal with the pressures of work, kids, and her anxiety about going out. And nothing stands in the way of her quest to become even more fit. "Losing the weight, finding time to eat healthy and work out, dealing with all the pressures in life—it's all doable," Charla says. "And I'm proof it can be done!"

What about you? What exactly can you do about stress so you don't gain weight? Consider doing something other than just "getting through it." To start this process, you have to be aware of the stress in your life. You may want to write down all the things in the last two weeks that stressed you out: dealing with your in-laws, your youngest child wanting those $175 sneakers, your boss changing a deadline, the traffic on the way to work, your jeans feeling a bit tighter this morning, standing in line in security when your flight leaves in 30 minutes, being laid off and not knowing how you're going to pay your bills, and so forth.

Next, cross out all the things on your list that are out of your control. Make your mind up to let go of things you can't control and to control or change the things you can. To help me with this, I carry the serenity prayer in my purse. This 25-word prayer, written by Professor Reinhold Niebuhr at Union Theological Seminary in New York, has helped many people regain balance in their lives: "God, grant me the serenity to accept the things I cannot change, courage to change the things I can, and wisdom to know the difference."

The "control, change, or let go" concept embedded in the serenity prayer is an important key to stress management. Many people spend a lot of time worrying about things over which they have no control: other people, places, or things. We have to use our thoughts to control our emotions and our actions, which is perhaps the most important ingredient to living a happy, healthy, and rewarding life.

Some things, like constant interruptions, you can control. You can let the interrupters know you are busy and don't have time to talk. You can turn off your cell phone or check and answer email only at certain times during the day.

Other stresses, like rush-hour traffic, are usually beyond your control. But there are some things about rush-hour traffic that you can personally change. If possible, take a different route or travel at a different time. If these changes are not possible, you have to change your attitude about the situation to lessen the stress. You can listen to music, educational CDs, or audio books. Rush hour traffic won't seem as frustrating because you'll be doing something to help keep your mind off the traffic and the other drivers. Accept the fact that you can't control the traffic, no matter how much you yell and gesture at other drivers.

Here are other decompressing actions you can take to stay cool under pressure:

BREATHE. When you begin to feel overwhelmed, stop for a few minutes and take some slow, deep breaths. Close your eyes and focus on your breath and move your eyes from side to side. Stimulating the optical nerve can relax the body and release tension in your shoulders. Breathing this way will calm you down, clear your mind of clutter, and allow you to think about what you need to do next instead of having 20 competing thoughts and feelings fighting for space in your mind.

If you are interacting other distressed people, taking a deep breath will help you detach from their stress and in turn calm them down. When you react to them by raising your voice, it only escalates the problem, and you will feel worse. Taking a few deep breaths will give you more of a sense of control so that their reactions won't control yours. When you start to experience stress-related physical symptoms—backaches,

STRETCH TO DESTRESS

CHEST STRETCH IN A DOORWAY
Hold on to a door frame, with your elbows at shoulder height. Gently lean forward to feel a good stretch across your chest. Hold this position for about 10 counts. Repeat the stretch at least two times.

NECK STRETCH
Relax your shoulders and slowly lean your ear down toward your shoulder. Gently roll your chin down toward the shoulder and then back up toward the sky. Inhale as you lower your chin and exhale as you raise it. Repeat this movement with five deep breaths on each side.

CHAIR STRETCH
Count backward from 20 and continue focused breathing while sitting tall in your chair. On count 15, slowly roll your body forward, and at count 5 slowly roll back upright, stacking the vertebrae one at a time as you sit tall.

ABDOMINAL STRETCH
Sit tall in your chair. Picture your belly inflating like a balloon as you breathe deeply into your core. Exhale the breath as the balloon deflates.

headaches, neck aches, tightness in your jaw—deep breathing will help your muscles relax and release the tension in your body.

MEDITATION. Meditation is the practise of focusing your mind on positive energies. The first time I meditated, I kept wondering if I was doing it correctly. Truthfully, when you focus your mind on positive thoughts, there is no wrong way to do it. Set your timer for a minute, then three, then five. Focus your mind on positive thoughts or the problem that is causing you stress. Imagine inhaling white light (positive thoughts) and exhaling brown air (negative thoughts). One of my meditations goes like

STRETCH TO DESTRESS (continued)

On the next breath, widen your chest as you inhale and inflate the balloon. As you exhale, allow the balloon to once again deflate while you lower your shoulders and rib cage. Let your chin drop toward your chest. Repeat one more time and exaggerate the movements. Breathe more deeply by squeezing your shoulder blades together on the inhale and squeezing your chest inward on the exhale.

STANDING PINWHEEL
Standing with your arms and feet wide, rotate your body from your hips and twist gently back and forth. Breathe with the movement and allow your body to swing gently. While rotating, allow your arms to swing around and bend at the elbow to tap your shoulder or hip. Light tapping helps stimulate key pressure points on the body.

TAPPING
With one hand, tap with your fingertips up the opposite arm from your wrist up to your neck and then back down again two to three times. Repeat with the opposite hand. Then tap your chest and rib cage and then down each leg. The vibration energizes the muscles and skin and allows your body to relax.

this. Inhale: power, kindness, confidence, strength. And I say these words silently to myself. Exhale: guilt, fear, anxiety.

STRETCH YOUR BODY. Experts note that exercise is effective in burning the excess cortisol and other stress hormones such as adrenaline that fuel feelings of anxiety and stress. Exercise also releases endorphins, the body's natural chemicals that block anxiety and pain. A great form of stress-relieving exercise is stretching. The simple stretches in the box on pages 230–231 will increase circulation and release upper back tension. Perform them whenever you need to ease anxiety.

TAI CHI. Tai chi is a system of movements designed to reduce stress and enhance health and longevity. It teaches you to be aware of where your body is tense. Through practice, you learn how to relax your mind and body so that inner pressure is replaced with inner peace. Try some basic tai chi rocking movements: Inhale as you take both hands up to chest height and push the air in front of you to the right and lean into the right side of the body. Exhale as you hold your body, shoulders, and head to the side. Then repeat to the other side. Perform 10 breaths.

DIET DESTRESSORS. When you're stressed, avoid foods that stress out your body such as caffeine and sugar. Eat more fresh fruits and vege-tables and drink lots of water. Fruits and vegetables are chock-full of nutrients, including the antioxidants your body needs to fight the harmful effects of free radicals and possibly combat cortisol's negative effects.

TAKE A MULTI. Stressed people tend to have poor diets, so taking a multi-vitamin and mineral supplement as an insurance policy makes sense.

ORGANIZE AND PRIORITIZE TASKS. Many people are overscheduled and therefore overwhelmed. Revisit your Charting My Day log in Appendix H to look at where you might still be wasting time. Then list the tasks you need to accomplish and sort them in the following categories: urgent, important, necessary, and not necessary. Work on the urgent and impor-tant tasks first, get them done, and you'll feel a greater sense of control over your life. Try saying "no" to at least one extra commitment a day to increase your sense of control and keep you from defaulting to negative coping strategies.

PROBLEM-SOLVE. Stressful situations usually do not resolve themselves. You have to take some sort of action. Let's say you're in debt over your head, and the situation is driving you to eat. Solving the problem might involve working with a financial counselor to set up a debt repayment plan or changing your personal spending behaviors to avoid debt in the future. We can eliminate, reduce, or alter some stressful aspects of our lives to lessen their impact. Whatever the problem, there's always a solution. Try to isolate exactly what is making you feel stressed. Brainstorm all possible solutions and options without judgment, and then narrow the solutions down to the most workable and the most effective. Act on them and evaluate how they worked.

GET A PET. People with pets not only live longer, happier lives, but pets can help us destress by providing company and unconditional love. Engage with your pet by trying Paws-ilates™, explained on pages 234–235.

RECAST YOUR STRESS. Think of a situation that recently caused you a great deal of anxiety. Describe the event in writing, but rewrite it with a happier ending, with a better solution, or with other options for handling it. This exercise will give you the confidence and options to deal with this type of situation in the future so that it induces less stress. Writing can reduce levels of cortisol, which can inhibit your body's natural defenses and make you fat if levels are too high.

VISUALIZE. Picture the stress that burdens you as a small flame in front of you. Breathe slowly to blow the flame out.

EMPOWER YOURSELF. Create an empowerment card with phrases on it such as:

I deserve to be happy and successful.
My body is dynamic and has the ability to heal and find its perfect weight.
My body is a beautiful gift to be respected and nourished.
I have the power to make the healthiest choices for myself.
I am becoming strong and fit every day.

Words of empowerment will fortify your commitment to the Naked Fitness program. If you want a daily or weekly empowerment emailed to you free of charge, go to my website and sign up for this service at www.nakedfitnesshealth.com.

PAW-ILATES™: A PUPPY UPPER

Research has linked pet ownership with lower blood pressure and choles-terol levels, better psychological well-being, reduced stress and loneliness, and increased longevity after a heart attack. Spending time with your pet definitely lowers stress, which in turn strengthens your immune system.

As the owner of two dogs, I have created Paws-ilates™. It blends spine-strengthening exercises, core toners, and some simple lifts with Fido, or in my case, Wrigley, to help you stand taller and spend time with your dog. Here are a few simple exercises I recommend with dogs that weigh 25 pounds or less.

SIT, LEAN, AND REACH

Start in a seated position on the floor, with knees slightly bent. Your pooch sits in front and facing you. Holding onto your pet with both hands, lean back and reach. Simply secure your pet, engage your core and lean back and reach. Keep your spine tall and chest open. Exhale as you lean back; inhale as you sit upright. Perform 10 to 20 alternating repetitions.

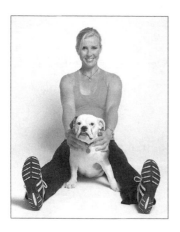 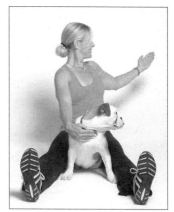

PAW-ILATES™: A PUPPY UPPER (continued)

CANINE CROSS

Start in a seated position with knees slightly bent with pet held securely. Rotate to the left side and return to center seated upright. Repeat to the right side. Lift the same side leg that you are turning toward to challenge your core.

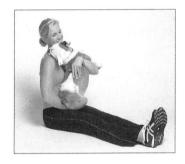 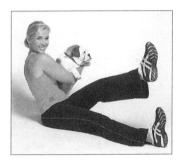

SIDE BEND POWER LEASH

Stand tall with your dog seated at your side. As you hold the leash with one hand and a bent arm, lift your other arm up and over your head. Reach downward toward your pet. Perform 10 repetitions and then walk your dog in a circle to repeat on the other side.

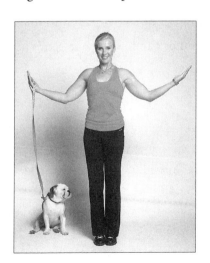 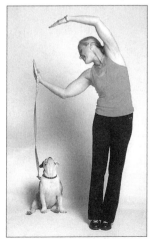

STRESS-RELIEVING MANTRAS

- Accept that some days you're the pigeon, and some days you're the statue.

- Always keep your words soft and sweet, just in case you have to eat them.

- If you lend someone $20 and never see that person again, it was probably worth it.

- It may be that your sole purpose in life is simply to be kind to others.

- Never put both feet in your mouth at the same time, because then you won't have a leg to stand on.

- Nobody cares if you can't dance well. Just get up and dance.

- When everything's coming your way, you're in the wrong lane.

- Birthdays are good for you. The more you have, the longer you live.

- Ask yourself these four questions: Why? Why not? Why not me? Why not now?

- Many of our dreams at first seem impossible, then they seem improbable, and only when we summon them will they will become inevitable.

- Don't be pushed by your problems. Be led by your dreams.

- Success is a ladder that you cannot climb with your hands in your pockets.

STAY GRATEFUL. In your journal, record everything you are grateful for. This practice helps you understand all that is wonderful and positive in your life and will restore a state of calmness and appreciation in your life. Give yourself credit every day. Each day, take a moment to pat yourself on the back for all the things you did. This will shift your perspective, helping you appreciate the great balancing act you pull off daily—working, parenting, volunteering, maintaining a social life, caring for elders, and so forth.

Stress tends to derail a healthy living program, but only if you let it. From this point forward, practice at least one of these stress-relieving techniques each day. The afternoon is the best time because this is when our bodies churn out the highest levels of cortisol.

With as many obstacles stripped away as possible, there's no stopping you in your quest to get fit and healthy—and stay that way.

14

STRIP AWAY: EMOTIONAL OVEREATING

Does a fight with your mate or an argument with your teenager propel you straight to the bottom of an ice-cream carton? Does an impending job interview send you to the nearest drive-through lane faster than you can say, "Fries with that, please"? Did you have a flat tire on the way home from work and then make a beeline to the fridge? Perhaps you eat when you're tense, lonely, afraid, depressed, or angry—pretty much any time things go a bit wrong. If so, you may be overeating in response to emotions such as boredom, loneliness, anger, sadness, or fear. Food becomes an outlet for you whenever you feel out of sorts.

You are not alone. I often see clients who are committed to losing weight, but as soon as they get into a fight with their husband or have a bad day at work, they'll plow through a whole box of cookies. From a very young age, we're taught to use food as a psychological coping mechanism. It's a reward if we've done well or a comfort if we've had a tough day.

Women are particularly susceptible because they're conditioned from childhood to suppress certain feelings, so they use food as a form of self-soothing. Research shows that the top foods overeaten by females are ice cream, chocolate, and cookies. These sweets temporarily elevate your level of serotonin (a feel-good hormone) and lower the level of cortisol (a stress hormone).

Liz J., one of my clients, knows what a powerful opponent emotional overeating can be. She had been overweight most of her adult life and packed on pounds with each of her four pregnancies over 10 years. "Food controlled almost every aspect of my life. I often ate because I was bored or upset, not because I was truly in need of nourishment. I never exercised and often used food to stuff down any pleasant or unpleasant feelings and emotions. If I was happy, I ate. If I was sad, I ate. If I was bored, I ate. Anything sweet, fried, or starchy had an anesthetic effect, and I felt calmer, happier, and less anxious after I ate. Eventually, the emotional overeating led to a weight gain of around 160 pounds, which left me feeling miserable and hopeless. I had little energy for any activity. As the years passed, I developed type 2 diabetes, hypertension, and elevated cholesterol. I felt miserable about the way I looked and felt."

Liz knew she had to change her relationship with food. Writing in her journal, she began to evaluate what she ate, when she ate, and what triggered the overeating. Patterns started to emerge. She was overeating to numb painful emotions.

"I decided I didn't have any option but to lose weight. I began a low-fat diet. I shopped for healthier foods like chicken, fruit, vegetables, oatmeal, and other whole grains. I was thrilled when I had lost 9 pounds the first week of eating in a more healthy fashion.

"I also ate meals on smaller plates or spread my food out over the plate so it looked like I was eating more food than I really was. I knew I would get used to eating less.

"When it came to exercise, I walked four to five times a week for 30 minutes and each week increased the intensity and distance. Eventually, I started strength training a few times a week."

Tackling the emotional overeating, however, was a challenge. Liz learned to use relaxation techniques such as meditating, journal writing, and just talking about her feelings. These actions were much more effective and healthier ways to handle her emotions than overeating. Over several years, she slowly replaced her destructive behavior from the past with more healthy habits.

She continued to eat well and to exercise under her doctor's supervision. Continuing with her healthy habits, Liz reached her goal weight of 130 pounds three years later.

"I stopped rewarding good behavior choices with food," she added. "One day, I put on my prom dress from 30 years ago—and it fit! I couldn't believe it. In all honesty, it fits me better now than it did back then."

In the past, Liz and her husband would vacation with their daughters at amusement parks in Florida. To her embarrassment, she'd have to sit on the sidelines because she was so overweight. Once Liz reached her goal weight, she returned with her family to Florida. "I'm proud to say I rode every ride that I could not ride before."

As a part of her journey, she learned the importance of eating as a fuel source for her body instead of an emotional cure-all. Liz found that when she ate healthy foods, she felt better.

"People always ask me what they should eat or how much weight they should lose. I tell them I believe in the 3 Ds of success: desire, determination, and discipline. Losing weight takes all three. Once they're in place, the rest will follow."

Today, Liz is training for a 5K race (she's 50). When she achieves that goal, she wants to run another race, maybe a half marathon.

"Looking back, I realize that I not only have changed how my body looks, but I also have changed the way I think of my body. I take time each day to nurture myself and surround myself with positive-thinking people, especially my husband and family. I don't focus on my body's flaws or wish to change any part of it. Instead, I've learned to love every muscle and curve.

"Losing weight and keeping it off can be a challenging and life-changing journey, but worth the energy it takes. Motivation can be sometimes hard to maintain, but if you dream and believe, you will achieve. I did!"

I'm sure you can relate to Liz's experience if you are an emotional overeater. But are you really? Take the quiz on pages 242–243 to find out.

ARE YOU AN
EMOTIONAL OVEREATER?

Take this short quiz to find out.

1. I turn to food when I'm sad, disappointed, or lonely.
    Yes _____   No _____

2. I often eat past the point of fullness.
    Yes _____   No _____

3. When I'm upset, I crave sweets or salty snack foods.
    Yes _____   No _____

4. When I go to parties or dine out with friends, I tend to overeat.
    Yes _____   No _____

5. If I eat too much, I feel guilty afterwards.
    Yes _____   No _____

6   I eat more than I should when I'm home alone or bored.
    Yes _____   No _____

7. My moods have the biggest influence on when and how I eat.
    Yes _____   No _____

8. I like to nurture family and friends with food.
    Yes _____   No _____

9. I think about food a lot.
    Yes _____   No _____

10. I am unhappy with my weight, but I overeat anyway.
    Yes _____   No _____

11. Eating is my favorite activity.
    Yes _____   No _____

12. I tend to clean my plate; I don't like to waste food.
    Yes _____   No _____

ARE YOU AN
EMOTIONAL OVEREATER? (continued)

13. I binge habitually.

Yes _____   No _____

14. The large amount of food I eat embarrasses me.

Yes _____   No _____

15. Sugary foods tend to calm me down.

Yes _____   No _____

SCORING

Count up your yeses and your noes.

If you answered yes to eight or more questions:

Your feelings of anger, frustration, loneliness, sadness, boredom, or even happiness might be causing you to overeat. And you are probably an emotional overeater. You may be eating too much or eating chaotically, but what you are really feeding is something in your life: relationship problems, broken dreams, financial worries, or problems at work. Try the strategies in this chapter, but don't be afraid to seek professional help.

If you answered yes to four to seven questions:

You may be struggling with some emotions from time to time. You are a borderline emotional overeater. At this point, it will be easier to get your eating habits under control by applying some of the strategies in this chapter.

If you circled three or fewer yeses:

You probably aren't an emotional overeater. You may occasionally use food to cope, but for the most part, it doesn't interfere with your ability to manage your weight.

If you are an emotional overeater or have tendencies toward it, you have to strip away emotional overeating to say fit and healthy. Here are the strategies to help you do that.

Analyze Your Eating Patterns

Work on understanding the emotions that are triggering your overeating: Anger? Anxiety? Loneliness? Frustration? Boredom? Fatigue? Spiritual emptiness?

If we could better manage these eating triggers, we'd all probably be a lot more slender. Unfortunately, it is not that easy, since our urges to eat are often more neurological than nutritional. Telling someone who is very reactive to food to stop eating is like saying to them, "Stop breathing," because food is a very powerful drive—more powerful in some people than in others.

It can be helpful to monitor your eating. Writing down not only what you eat, but also the circumstances under which you ate (time, place, who you were with, your emotional state, or other events such as a fight with your spouse). Do you eat when someone criticizes your work or your parenting? Or when the clock is ticking on a major project? Keeping track makes you aware of your patterns and gives you an opportunity to make better choices.

In addition, ask yourself, "What am I really hungry for?" Before eating chips, a candy bar, or cookies, listen to both your body and your emotions. Are you physically hungry, or is something else going on? If your "hunger" isn't physical, see if you can find ways to feed those needs that don't involve eating.

The Naked Fitness Food Journal in Appendix I will walk you through this process. At the end of the week, read over your record and look for patterns. What were the events, people, places, or situations that led to the emotional eating?

Apply Solutions

Once you know your triggers, you can pinpoint the solutions that will work for you. If your journal reveals that you eat when you're bored or stressed, for example, find other ways to distract or calm yourself in those situations. Here are some suggestions.

MEDITATE

Several minutes of meditation coupled with deep breathing can stop a binge in its tracks. Employ your mantras or pray. Ask for peace and calm. Remind yourself that you can do this. Repeat your mantra or prayer until the emotion passes.

INTERRUPT THE URGE

People usually give in because they've never let themselves ride the wave of their urges to binge. They give in as the crest of the urge is still building. The trick, then, is to surf that crest and get past it. Distract yourself in ways that get you away from food. Hop into the car—minus spare change for the convenience store—or run an errand. Instead of watching TV after dinner, which may trigger snacking, pick up the phone and call a friend. Get yourself doing something other than thinking, "I want food, I want food!"—anything to get your mind off food. If you're successful at "urge surfing," the desire to binge will pass.

EXERCISE INSTEAD OF OVEREATING

Take a walk, practice yoga, or work out. Ten minutes can be enough to feel refreshed. Exercise naturally lifts mood by boosting endorphins and serotonin levels, and that boosts your mood and leaves you feeling less anxious.

Other ways to get back in emotional balance include:

- Embracing the feeling: accepting it and letting it fade
- Expressing it: talking, writing, praying
- Learning from it: asking yourself, "What could I have done differently?"

- Developing a plan: asking yourself, "How will I approach this?"
- Meeting the need logically: If you're angry and upset, express it constructively; if you're tired, sleep; if you're lonely, call a friend; if you're restless, take a walk; if you're truly hungry, eat

THINK BEFORE YOU EAT

Before you eat that pint of ice cream, ask, "Is this really what I need? Will this make me feel better?" Think about how you'll feel after you binge: bloated, lethargic, and ashamed. Is that how you want to feel? Eventually you'll learn to say, "I love myself too much to keep treating myself like this."

LEAN ON SOMEONE

Sometimes what we need to circumvent a lapse into emotional overeating is support. If that's the case, call a friend or talk to your partner. If this is hard for you, you need to learn to ask others for help. Don't expect people to read your mind and know what you need. This may require learning how to be assertive rather than waiting for someone to notice.

It may be helpful to seek group or one-on-one therapy to further explore the issues that provoke your tendency to overeat.

PLACES

Locales, certain rooms in our homes, or our cars can also be triggers associated with emotional overeating. I have some suggestions:

- If driving home from work takes you by your favorite drive-through, find another route.
- If you overeat or snack in front of the television, make it a rule in your house to always eat in the dining room.
- If you're vulnerable to over-snacking the moment you walk in the front door after work, revamp your daily diet so that you're less ravenous. Make sure to eat a healthy, filling snack at mid-morning and mid-afternoon, and don't skip lunch. Or instead of raiding the fridge after coming home, do your exercise routine and squeeze in a walk.

MANAGE BOREDOM

If you really have nothing to do, choose a snack that requires time and energy, such as microwave popcorn, unshelled nuts, even crunchy foods like carrots that involve a lot of chewing. These types of foods force you to eat slowly and be more conscious of how much you're putting in your mouth. They also take a while to eat, so they help pass the time without filling you up with fattening calories.

TACKLE DEPRESSION

While it's perfectly normal for you mood to occasionally dip, ongoing depression can interfere with your ability to get things done, including workouts and weight control. If you find a bad mood getting in the way of productive living, by all means, consult a psychologist or psychiatrist for help.

In addition, there are some natural forms of relief you can try. Exercise, of course, is one of the best ways to lift your spirits. Also, get a daily dose of vitamins and sun. Together, these strategies can help banish the blues. Researchers at the University of Washington School of Nursing asked 112 women who were mildly to moderately depressed to walk briskly outside for 20 minutes and take five micrograms of folic acid, 400 IU of vitamin D, and 200 micrograms of selenium. The women also increased their exposure to bright light, both natural and artificial, during the day. After eight weeks, almost all the women reported feeling less depressed, and 25 percent had lost weight, even though they had not been dieting. Many of the women were eating less at meals and snacking less. They even mentioned that their cravings for carbs had diminished.

CELEBRATE WITH FOOD—IN MODERATION

It's perfectly fine to celebrate with food, as long as you don't go overboard and stuff yourself silly. One of the pleasures of eating is enjoying food with friends and celebrating good times.

That doesn't mean you always have to celebrate with food. The next time something fabulous happens invent a new kind of feel-good ritual. Instead of treating yourself to a special dinner with your husband, take an afternoon off and spend it with him. To recognize your daughter's accomplishment, join her in an activity like skating or biking. Rather than celebrate your birthday at the office, ask your coworkers to take a walk with you in place of eating cake and ice cream. Begin to retrain your brain to celebrate without food.

ENJOY FOOD

Along those same lines, don't try to substitute chopped celery when you really want a few nachos. Trying to deprive yourself of certain foods all the time will backfire and trigger binges on those very foods. Learn how to eat smaller portions of "nondiet" foods. If you can't eat just one handful of chips, don't buy large bags. Purchase single-serving sizes instead. Or if your favorite indulgence is chocolate, keep it out of the house. Instead, go to an expensive candy store on occasion and treat yourself to just a single serving of chocolate.

Eat a variety of foods in moderation; this will put a lid on your desire to overeat. Fill up on high-fiber foods too. They take up a lot of space in your tummy, so you're less likely to gorge on them.

And remember, not all comfort foods are necessarily fattening or bad for you. Whole grains, for example, contain an amino acid that helps boost a mood-elevating chemical in the brain. Lean proteins such as chicken, tuna, and turkey have another type of amino acid that helps boost energy and helps the body cope better with emotions. As you become more practiced at handling difficult feelings instead of eating through them, you'll eat more for fuel than comfort. In short, a healthy diet, rich with natural foods, can positively affect your behavior and energy levels.

Stripping away the cycle of emotional overeating could be one of the most important actions you'll ever take. It will ease feelings of guilt about food and give you a new faith in your ability to look after yourself with compassion. You'll also learn more about who you are and love who you are, even when naked.

15

STRIP AWAY: SABOTEURS

It could be your spouse, you mother, your best friend. They know you're trying to eat right and exercise regularly, but then comes the pound of chocolate candy on Valentine's Day, the carry-out pizza with everything on it, the invitation to an all-you-can-eat pancake breakfast.

There's no doubt about it. One of the biggest stumbling blocks to eating healthfully and getting fit is having a circle of friends, colleagues, and family members who do not, and who may even sabotage your attempts to lose weight by teasing you about your diet.

How can you stick to your fitness commitment when you're surrounded by saboteurs—people who knowingly or unknowingly may be undermining your fitness efforts? Here are my recommendations for stripping away saboteurs.

Turn Saboteurs in to Supporters

Some saboteurs may feel threatened by your decision to get into shape. A good example is the wife who loses a lot of weight. Her husband frets over whether he'll lose her to another man, so he tries to fatten her up again. To him, life was more secure when lived in the old patterns. The feeling of being threatened is very real.

So is jealously. Your best friend might feel jealous of your success at losing weight—a feeling that drives a wedge in your relationship. Granted, those emotions are not your problem, and you should not shift your course to win the approval of others. But it's good to be sensitive to their feelings, particularly those of a spouse or close friend.

Ultimately, those who are unsupportive of your fitness efforts may not be attacking you but trying to deal with their own issues. You can lessen their impact on your life by taking the time to understand them better.

Another good strategy is to turn the saboteur into a supporter.

You might invite your spouse, friend, or family member to try exercising or a new healthy food for a trial period. Your invitation might go something like this to a spouse" "I want to spend more time with you because I love being together. Let's try an exercise program together, just for two weeks to see how we like it." Or to a friend or loved one: "I'd like to stay in touch with you more often. Why don't we join an exercise class or walk together in the morning to keep each other motivated?"

By sharing the experience with a partner, you can help each other stay motivated. Partners encourage one another to move from unhealthy to healthy behaviors. And I know from experience with my clients that people who work out with their spouses or friends are more likely to stick to their fitness programs than those who go it alone.

Sharing the fitness experience gives you both something new to talk about together, and better communication is always a source of greater closeness. At the end of the trial period, you could give your partner some type of fitness gift such as a new warm-up suit or a gift certificate for athletic shoes. By that time, hopefully, your partner will want to join you in continuing this powerful new lifestyle.

Ask for or Find Support

If you recognize your saboteurs in advance, you can recruit most of the people around you to support, rather than derail, your diet. If you communicate your need for support, chances are people will provide it.

Connecting with other people who are like-minded, have positive goals, and encourage you to reach your goals not only provides valuable support, but it will also give you a network of people who will hold you accountable for the goals that you have set. Ellie, 45, grew up overweight, stashing food under her bed and eating in private—rarely, if ever, socializing. Eventually, her weight ballooned to 200 pounds.

"I was well on my way to 250 pounds and all the extras that come along with it: diabetes, heart disease, and breathing problems," she told me.

Ellie felt totally isolated. Then she heard about the Naked Fitness groups I was starting, and she signed up to be in group 1. There she met other people just like her—an experience that changed her life. "I was welcomed with open arms," she remembered. Finding supportive friends made all the difference in her weight-loss success. In no time at all, she lost 30 pounds, and she credits the group with the inspiration to get her going.

"I'm now looking forward to not clothes-shopping in the 'more of a woman' section," she said proudly. "And I'm ready to start tucking my shirt in again."

When you get involved with a group or form a new relationship, it has the power to change you and change your life. I see this all the time in my weekly Naked Fitness support groups, where participants gather to exercise, talk, and bond, because they share something in common—a desire to lose weight and renew their health. Being with like-minded individuals is a wonderful way to enhance your energy.

Whenever possible, enlist buddies with similar experiences. If you're looking for people who can help you eat right and exercise, some of the most inspiring supporters will be those who've been there, done that. Make sure the people on your list bring positive, upbeat, and inspiring energy to your efforts.

You could even create your own group. This could be as simple as forming a walking club, inviting your friends over to do your Naked Fitness workouts, or sharing insights into using Naked Fitness principles with your group.

Plan Ahead

It's easier to stick to a healthy course of action if you decide to do so before the saboteurs present themselves. I practice this principle often. If I'm watching my diet, I make a pact with myself that I will not eat things that could compromise that goal. Preplanning works much better than merely throwing caution to the wind.

Or suppose you're sticking to your plan but are invited to an event where all the "wrong" foods will be served. Graciously ask permission to bring some of your own food or politely explain to your host or hostess your reasons for not eating certain foods.

Use Assertive Dialogue

You have to be clear and direct about what you want in order to get helpful support. Let's say you've started working out and eating more healthfully. After being overweight for most of your adult life, you've lost almost 50 pounds and are at a healthy weight. But your mom keeps telling you you're too thin and accuses you of having an eating disorder. Let's face it, Mom still thinks you're a growing guy or gal who needs to eat. It isn't that Mom wants to make you fat. She just equates food with love. The more of her homemade spaghetti you scarf down, the more loved she feels.

How can you win?

Respond to your mother from an adult position. Say something along the lines of, "You know that I've been to my doctor," or "I've spoken to my nutritionist [or my trainer], and my weight and eating habits are healthy."

After that, state what you need from her. "I really am working hard. I'm feeling great, and it would be nice to have your support. Is there anything I can do to help you give me that?"

If that doesn't work, set certain boundaries. Tell your mother that when you see her, certain topics are off-limits, such as food, eating habits, weight, and your body.

There are other strategies you can use for anyone who pushes food on you by offering you food that's not on your plan. Rather than giving in because you don't want to offend anyone, say, "Not just yet, I'm going to wait a while." This is probably enough to convince most people that you'll eat eventually, so they'll leave you alone.

Worried about hurting the cook's feelings? "Thank you, I won't be having any of those today and I really appreciate the time you took to make them," said in a confident, loving tone gets across the point without causing hurt. You can be kind and considerate and take care of yourself at the same time.

Try praising the food pushers, too. When seconds are offered, don't say you're on a diet. It sometimes signals hosts to push harder. Instead, try one of these lines: "Your dinner was so delicious and I enjoyed it so much, I don't have room for another bite." Or: "I'm so full, but I'd love to take dessert home for later." (But toss it out after you get home!)

With some people, a firm "No, thank you" may be all that's necessary. Kindness and tact go a long way when you're turning down somebody's "masterpiece" dish or special-occasion cookies.

Begin to plan your responses to the pressure to eat more. Arm yourself with a few simple replies such as, "You're right, one piece of cheesecake won't hurt me, but it won't help me reach my goals either," or "I'm saving my calories for a second glass of wine." With a little practice, you will get comfortable verbalizing your thoughts and goals without feeling scrutinized or pressured.

You can also share your eating records with your spouse, your mom, or other loved ones and explain which eating habits you're working on, such as cutting back on sweets and eating more fruits and veggies. These help your saboteurs understand and accept your goals. Explain what you need in terms of support in a way that doesn't put anyone on the defensive, such as: "I appreciate you bringing home dinner, but I need you to respect my desire to eat healthier and not surprise me with fattening food."

Another tactic is to write your family and friends a letter asking them for support. Talk about your goals and how they can support you. Point out behaviors that drive you to cheat and ask for their encouragement.

Learn to communicate to a partner, loved one, friend, or family member who may not support your fitness goals by standing up for yourself, asking for support, planning ahead, and keeping a positive, upbeat attitude about your new lifestyle.

Have a Contest

Band together at work to lose weight, and make it competitive. On-the-job dieting is a great weight-control tool, and your employer will probably be supportive if they're worried about health insurance costs. A trimmer workforce could mean lower medical expenses and higher productivity for the employer. The competitive nature of the business environment is a good motivator.

Some employers let workers run the competitions without formal support or intervention. Others may give out prizes, offering lower health care premiums for employees who participate in a company weight-loss program or providing discounts on an independent weight-loss program.

These contests can promote teamwork and cooperation among employees. It's fun when you've got more people to support you. Having 20 or 30 of your closest friends and colleagues doing it with you it makes it easier. It's spreading. It's contagious. It creates a sense of camaraderie, and you get a sense of accomplishment on a weekly basis.

Guard against Group Overeating

The power of people, particularly groups, to influence our behavior negatively is more common and subtle than you might think. (I'm not talking about your support people here, but rather those who can be bad influences.) When we're in a group, we want to fit in, so we try to conform to the group behavior. A group can be a work group, a bunch of friends, neighbors, and so forth. Because many group activities center around eating and drinking, you have to be on your guard to not fall in with unhealthy group behaviors.

If certain people or groups tend to trigger unhealthy habits in your life, here are some strategies to consider:

- If you're going to dinner with a group of friends and are concerned you'll overeat, eat some natural high-fiber foods (such as raw veggies or fresh fruit) before you go. You'll be less likely to pig out later.

- Have a good exercise session or long walk the day of the gathering. On exercise days, I've found that I'm less likely to undo the beneficial effects of my workout by splurging.

- Try to arrange social activities that don't include food, such as going to the movies, a concert, or play.

Build Support from Knowledgeable Professionals

Working with a qualified registered dietician or trainer is another way of building support. An RD can help you plan meals, and trainers can give you the right workout advice for your situation.

You'll want to make sure you select certified trainers who are well informed, experienced, and dependable. Ask your gym, your doctor, or your friends for names. Make appointments with these professionals to discuss your goals.

If you're looking for a trainer, determine who has certified this individual. The website www.fitnessconnect.com will link you with a professional trainer in your area who is certified by the most reputable organizations in the world.

Ask for references from other clients, medical professionals, or both who are familiar with the trainer's or nutritionist's abilities and skills. Take the time to follow up on these referrals. Your efforts may save you future grief.

Once you look into these areas, find out what his or her fitness philosophy is. This information may help you develop a clear idea of what you're getting yourself into before you hand over any money.

Because they need to establish your baseline fitness levels, medical conditions, and nutritional habits, an experienced professional will almost always have a slew of tests and paperwork ready for you to fill out before you begin any type of regimen.

Another important factor is interpersonal skills. If you're a client looking for a professional, you should have a very good feeling about how you interact and how you communicate. It's all about trying to find someone whose personality meshes well with yours.

FRIEND-ILATES™ FOR EXTRA SUPPORT

Try my Friend-ilates™ exercises to help you stick with your fitness program. The exercises in this Friend-ilates™ partner training routine will build muscle, burn calories, and strengthen your friendship.

PASS TO YOUR PARTNER

Stand back to back, one of you holding a medicine ball, barbell, or large phone book (anything that weighs about six to eight pounds). Keep your knees slightly bent and pass the object to your partner in a clockwise direction for 8 to 10 reps and switch directions. This will strengthen your core muscles, shoulders, and biceps.

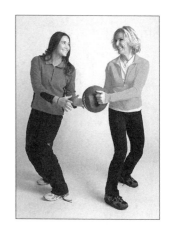

SIT, REACH, AND PASS

Start seated side by side with a medicine ball, barbell, or large phone book (anything that weighs about six to eight pounds). Lean slightly back off your "sits bones" onto the soft part of your backside and pass the weighted object to your partner. Lift your arms over head and lift one leg (keep both feet on the ground if you need to).

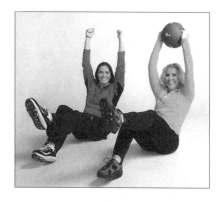

Pass the weight back to your partner. Aim for 8 to 10 reps with your partner on your left, and then switch sides. This move borrows from Pilates core moves with weight-training waist rotations, which results in a tight midsection and great shoulders.

FRIEND-ILATES™ FOR EXTRA SUPPORT (continued)

THE HOOKUP

Start seated side by side with both knees bent to the outside. Hook elbows to help balance each other and keep your chests lifted and your posture tall. Lift and lower the back leg. Aim for 12 to 15 repetitions on each side, and then turn around and repeat on the other leg. This exercise builds a better backside and strengthens the core and spinal muscles. Use your partner for stability and balance, and keep those elbows lifted to work the shoulders.

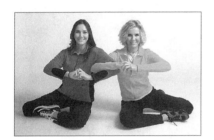 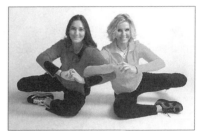

PARTNER PUSH

This one may look easy, but it's really intense. Start standing and facing one another, and extend your arms out in front of you. Keeping your arms extended, one partner pushes against the other partner's hands. Both of you are providing resistance and pressing against the other. You will feel this in the backs of your arms but also your abs and midsection. Hold for 10 seconds and then switch sides, still facing each other. Alternate the direction of push for a set of 10.

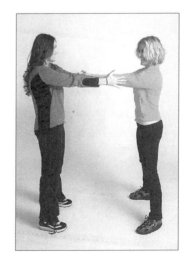

FRIEND-ILATES™ FOR EXTRA SUPPORT (continued)

PARTNER SQUATS

Lean on your friend in this squat exercise to build trust and tone your legs and butt. Start back to back and slowly lower yourselves to a sitting position. Lift your crossed arms to improved your posture and strengthen your shoulders. Try to hold at the bottom for five counts and return to a standing position. Aim for 12 to 15 repetitions. This exercise really works the legs and helps improve balance.

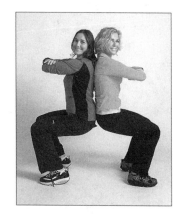

BALLET CROSS REACH

This stretch and balance move feels amazing. Start with elbows hooked standing about 12 to 18 inches apart, side by side. Step your outside foot behind and grab hands over your heads. Pull your arms upward and press your hips out to the side. This opens the IT band, obliques, and lats, which become tight after most cardio exercise. Hold for 10 to 30 seconds and repeat on the other side. This is a great exercise after your walk or jog with a friend.

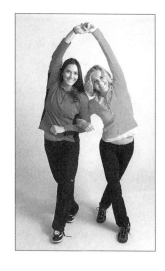

Be a Role Model

No matter how things turn out, be a fitness role model—flesh-and-blood proof that people can lose weight without being miserable—as well as a practical example of how to do it. Let people see that you enjoy food shopping, cooking, eating, and working out.

When you start to change right before people's eyes, this can inspire them to improve their own lives. Keep your commitment to a fit lifestyle. If your spouse and loved ones see consistency in your life, they're more likely to follow in your footsteps. You personal commitment and conviction can inspire others to follow your path.

Stripping away all these obstacles will help you stay in shape forever. Continue to concentrate on your diet and workout. Find activities you enjoy, and keep moving. Don't punish yourself; just take care of your health! If it seems boring sometimes, just look at yourself in the mirror and remind yourself how unhealthy you felt when you were overweight. The goal is to enjoy your new body—the one that now epitomizes Naked Fitness.

Be healthy and be moved!

Resources
and
Tools

Look Five Pounds Thinner in Five Minutes

So many people get caught in the trap of thinking, "I'll be happy when I lose 50 pounds, 75 pounds, 100 pounds," that they can't be satisfied until they arrive at their goal weight. This way of thinking makes it hard to achieve your goal and stay there because you delay happiness and self-satisfaction—a negative state of mind that makes you feel like a failure—and have no good energy to help you get to that goal. If you believe you can't be happy or satisfied until you are thin, you will be more likely to give up out of dissatisfaction and frustration with yourself.

But if you can say, "I eventually want to be thinner, but in the meantime I can be happy with myself and enjoy my body and my looks the way they are now," the energy around you will be magnetic, and you'll draw to you what you most desire: a beautiful, fit, healthy body.

This part of the book will teach you how to feel good—and thin—right now. I'll show you how to look 5 pounds thinner in five minutes and transform your physical appearance immediately. Your physical appearance is important and goes far below the surface level of your life. It makes a statement about who you are and how you feel about yourself. If you look frumpy, you feel frumpy. If you look terrible in your clothes, you feel terrible. If you don't feel good about the way you look, it is difficult to feel confident, energetic, or motivated. It's your appearance, and you need to be comfortable with it and feel good about it. The more attractive you can make yourself look, the more confidence you will exude. Nothing is sexier than confidence.

We've all done it: stared in the mirror and asked the same question. "Does this make me look fat?" To stop that kind of judgmental thinking and self-criticism, the solution is simple: Choose the right clothes. And the right clothes are those that deemphasize what you don't like—real or imagined—and highlight what you do.

When you learn how to dress in clothes that flatter your figure, even right now, you'll feel better about yourself. Clothes—the right clothes— have the power to give you the psychological lift that is vital to the work you'll be doing on the Naked Fitness program.

In a recent segment on the TODAY show, breast cancer survivors told their stories of how they felt better when dressed up with flattering clothes and prettied up with a makeover, even thought their physical ill-ness had not changed. Even when I'm suffering through a cold and look-ing at the dark circles under my eyes, when I put on a little moisturizer, makeup, and comfortable clothes, I feel like a million bucks.

We tend to clothe ourselves in how we feel. When ready to relax and chill, you might slip on soft cotton, jersey-style pants, a loose-fitting T-shirt, fluffy socks, and cozy slippers. When heading to a business meet-ing, you might put yourself in a fitted sport-coat, pressed, starched oxford shirt, slacks, and highly polished heels. Or for a night on the town, you might wear your funnest, sexiest little number.

I like to pack fun clothes for vacations. My friend Lynette would always comment, "What 'costumes' did you bring for this trip?" I'd always have a few stylized outfits to add fun to our vacations together over the years.

Dress for success is my motto for Naked Fitness, and I bet it's already operating in your life. Maybe you went to a party last weekend and had a wonderful time. You felt fabulous. Now think about it: What did you wear that night? Remember it, make a note of it, and wear it again. If you felt fabulous wearing red, don't wear blue the next time! If you wore a turtle-neck, try wearing that turtleneck again. Learn how clothes make you feel.

Clothed, you can delude yourself as much as you want and believe you're a sex god or goddess. But standing naked in the mirror is much tougher; flaws scream at you loud and clear. So while I want you to learn to appreciate your naked body, flaws and all, I want you to also appreciate your clothed body.

There are really only two kinds of clothes in the world: those that flatter your shape and those that don't. Here are my suggestions for choosing clothes that make you look slimmer and at your very best.

Master Monochromatic

Outfits that are one color or a range of one color (e.g., varying shades of greens or grays) from head to toe or are close in tone make you look slimmer instantly. This is termed "monochromatic dressing."

It works for several reasons. Color is the first thing most people notice about an outfit. Even someone who knows nothing about fashion will notice color. Also, dressing in one color creates a strong, unbroken vertical line that elongates the body. Put another way, monochromatic dressing helps avoid "breaks." A break is any place where the eye stops because of a change in color or texture. The fewer the breaks, the trimmer you look.

To accomplish this, avoid dividing your body into two distinct sections. A body divided is a shorter—and heavier-looking—body. A white blouse with a black skirt, for instance, divides the body right in half. But when you pop on a black jacket, you've got a strong, dark monochromatic outer silhouette.

Dressing in one color doesn't have to be boring. You can incorporate as many different textures into an outfit as you like, and you'll be surprised at the pizzazz and sophistication you'll add. Texture can lend as much as a second color to an outfit. For example, picture a soft suede jacket, wool flannel slacks, and a silk scarf. Even if all the colors were nearly identical, the variation in textures would give the outfit a rich, interesting dimension and relief from same-old, same-old.

Stick Mostly to Dark Neutrals

Although the monochromatic plan will work in every color of the rainbow, dark neutral colors make you look more slender than light colors. They may not be the most adventurous colors, but they are the most slimming. This is because dark neutrals absorb light and recede into the background, rather than reflect light and pop out, as brighter colors do. Plus, details and construction lines, such as seams and darts, are absorbed by the density of dark colors, leaving fewer lines to distract the eye. Take the light-colored blouses or shirts in your closet. In most cases, when you wear them, you can probably see the outlines of seams, shoulder pads, sometimes even your bra. Not so with dark colors. The darker the color, the more invisible the construction.

You don't have to wear dark neutrals exclusively—just the basic pieces: jackets, slacks, suits, and coats. If you want to add color, you can always do it with blouses, sweaters, scarves, and other accessories.

Wear Clothes That Accentuate Your Body Type

We all come in a variety of pleasing shapes and sizes, and so do clothes. By selecting clothes that flatter your body, you'll look better and feel better instantly. If you take nothing else away from this chapter, take the advice in this section. What follows are various body-type issues and how to fix them with your clothes.

Bottom Heavy

- Add some extra dimension on top. One way to do this is by wearing shoulder pads. (Don't worry whether they're fashionable. Just limit their size—never too broad or thick.) Another way is to wear scarves or shawls around your shoulders. They add dimension at the top for balance and direct the eye up.

- Keep your belt fairly loose at your waistline. The more you cinch your waist, the bigger your hips look. And your belts should be narrow.

- Try a tailored, structured suit with wide-leg trousers. Wear either cropped jackets with a loose trouser and heel or tops or jackets that hit just below the hip with narrower pants to create long lines. Avoid tops and jackets that end right at the hip—the widest part of the body. They will only accentuate that area.

- Minimize large hips and thighs with long nipped-in blazers that fall to mid-thigh or lower.

- Wear jeans with a slight bell-bottom flare. The effect will help balance out broad hips. No skinny jeans, though. They will only accentuate your hips and middle areas.
- Choose textures with vertical lines or ribs.

All of these solutions help redirect attention from the broadness below to the slimness above.

Overall Heavier Build

- Try wearing more scoop- or V-neck tops. These will help draw the eyes down the body, elongating your body and focusing around your neck and face.
- Avoid clingy dresses with loud graphic prints. Instead, try solid-color dresses with plunging necklines.
- Avoid belts; they cut your body in half and accentuate a round middle.
- Avoid boxy, baggy clothes. They just make you look larger.
- Wear tailored tops that nip in at the waist to make your midsection look smaller.

Stocky or Athletic Build

- Try a bias-cut dress. Because the fabric is cut and sewn diagonally, it drapes in a way that makes your body look curvier.
- Gravitate toward deeper neck lines (V or scoop).
- Wear fitted tops and tanks that are cut in at the shoulders.
- Go for skirts and shorts with shorter inseams and fitted bottoms.
- Dress yourself in opposites: either fitted pants with a looser top or a fitted top with looser pants.
- Wear heels to help elongate your body.
- Avoid tight clothes on top and on bottom together. They can make you look more stocky.
- Try tight long sleeves and low necklines to flatter small busts.
- Go for ruching, empire lines below your bust, and feminine details.

Large Bust

- Select simple seams, higher necklines, or cross-over or wrap tops.

- Stay away from large patterns.

- Avoid blouses and dresses with ruching.

- Select scoop and V-neck styles to elongate your appearance. If you wear turtlenecks or other high-neck tops, the top of your body will look like one large mass. Lowering your neckline with V-necks and scooped necklines helps create distinction and definition between the chest and the rest of the upper body.

- Wear racer-back tanks, to minimize bounce, over a fitted zip-up jacket.

- Try a belted shirtdress to play down a busty figure.

Short-Waisted

- Wear cargo-style dresses with waistbands and buttons on the upper half only. The distinction between top and bottom will help define your midsection.

- Add a belt to further the waist-lengthening effect.

Short Stature

- Consider empire-waist dresses; they shift focus to a higher point on your body, creating the illusion of height.

- Wear pants that nearly skim the ground or at least skim the heels of your shoes.

- Choose wide-leg slacks to balance a generous bottom half. And kick back in boot-cut jeans with a bit of stretch for a trimming effect.

- For a short neck, steer clear of high-neck tops, which make you look shorter and heavier. Instead, wear deep-cut tops and dresses for maximum neck exposure: V-necks, boatnecks, square cuts, and U shapes.

- Go for long scarves worn vertically (don't wrap them around your neck), long necklaces that drape below the neckline, and delicate earrings. If your hair is long wear it up to elongate your neck.

- Wear high heels whenever they're practical. High-heeled shoes grant you what genetics didn't: a taller body and sexy legs. Go as high as you can safely stand. But if you're not good at balancing, choose styles with more surface area, like chunky heels and wedges. Pair your tall heels with heel-grazing slacks for a sleeker silhouette. Wear your high heels with dresses and skirts for a flirty, ultra-feminine look.

Flabby Arms

- Avoid tight sleeves, which emphasize full arms.
- Choose dresses and tops with open necklines, halter styles, and off-the-shoulder ensembles to focus attention on your neck, collarbone, and shoulders.
- Go sleeveless only when necessary.

Be Choosy about Undergarments

Wearing some of the new body-slimming, body-shaping undergarments can make you look five pounds thinner in five minutes no matter what your problem areas or your current clothing size. Your family and friends will think you've lost weight, even though you started Naked Fitness only this morning. Chalk it up to the illusion of undergarments.

So many companies are making so many variations of slimming tops, bottoms, bras, and underwear that there is literally something for everyone.

Find Your Style

We all have certain styles, shapes, colors, and silhouettes that look either great, fair, or terrible. Most of us own too many clothes that do nothing for us. For some reason we think we need different styles, but the truth is we'd be much better off sticking to the few that really play up our assets.

Once you find what works for you, there's no reason to wear things that don't flatter just for variety's sake. For example:

- If you look better in skirts than pants, then the majority of your bottoms should be skirts (if your lifestyle permits).

- If V-necks are more flattering than scoop necks, why even have turtle-necks in your closet?
- If long jackets suit you better than short ones, skip the short ones.
- If you look fabulous in red, why wear beige?

You get the idea. Once you start thinking along these lines, you'll probably end up wearing just 20 percent of your existing wardrobe—like most of us do anyway.

My recommendation for women today is to go to the same store over and over to create a relationship with one of the sales personnel. If she knows you—and is honest—she'll tell you, "Mrs. Smith, I don't think that you should buy this outfit."

Watch Out for Physique-Hazardous Textures

Avoid these textures for the following reasons:

- Stiff garments disregard your shape and take on one of their own, which is likely to be square and boxy.
- Bulky fabrics add mass and, depending on the fabric, can add more than an inch to your frame all around. If you're heavy right now, avoid a fisherman's sweater, heavy corduroy slacks, or a layered baggy tunic.
- Don't shine. Shiny textures have reflective surfaces that absorb light and make you seem bigger. The more matte the fabric, usually the more flattering it will be.

If It Doesn't Fit, Get Rid of It

There is nothing worse than always having to tug at your clothes or be constantly adjusting. A key aspect of clothing is the fit!

When something fits well, it can make you look five pounds leaner—and ten times better. Clothes that are too big can make you look big, and clothes that are too small can make you look big. Here are some fit problems that can add pounds, so get rid of or steer clear of any of these:

- Tight waistbands. As the waist gets squeezed, bulges are created under the rib cage and on the top of the hip. It happens with skirts, pants, shorts, tights, and even pantyhose. A loose waistband doesn't squeeze;

it skims the waist and allows the garment to fall gracefully. If you can't slip a couple of fingers between you and the waistband, it's probably too tight. You'll actually feel slimmer when the waist fits properly.

- Crotches that pull. Those horizontal lines across the front of your pants near the crotch happen when pants are too small.

- Seams that pull or pucker anywhere on your body. This gives the impression that there is something big underneath making it happen. The same goes for stressed zippers and gaping buttons.

- Pants that cut up between the buttocks or stretch tightly across the butt or thighs. Tight jeans are a common culprit in this category.

- Skirts that curve in under the buttocks. Skirts look slimmest when they fall straight over your butt.

- Buttocks peeking out under your jacket. Jackets should generally reach the bottom of your buttocks.

- A hemline that falls at the wrong place. Short skirts are most flattering when they fall right around a certain part of the knee—that little part that goes in at the knee on the inside. If the skirt ends just above that indentation, you'll be surprised how long and lean your leg will look. If you have heavy legs, long skirts look better when they reach the narrowest part of the calf.

So buy clothes that fit, not clothes you wish you could fit into. Clothing that's too tight will make you look fat and feel like a stuffed sausage, and it will end up discouraging you.

And while you're thinning out clothes that don't fit, get rid of extra accessories. Women tend to wear too much of everything. Too much jewelry, too much hair, too much makeup. I'm a believer in taking a second look in the mirror just before leaving the house and removing something. Whatever is gone won't be missed!

Feel Good in Your Workout Clothes

Ever notice how most of us will go and buy that special outfit for the interview, dinner date, class reunion, or upcoming 5K? Workout apparel is no different than the other clothes hanging in your closet. Having the right outfit that not only looks good, but also makes you feel good is the key. Mental and emotional readiness take one a lot farther than physical readiness.

Are there certain fabrics that one should stay away from when exercising? You'll often hear people bash cotton, because when cotton gets wet, it stays wet. It also holds sweat and bacteria. A good option is clothes for exercise-minded people that are made with a special type of fabric that wipes sweat from the body.

Stay away from polyester, nylon, and anything that doesn't breath or whisk away moisture. Synthetic fabrics like these just plain stink when they get sweaty.

Here are some top technical fabrics to look for in workout apparel:

- **X-Static.** This all-natural fiber system incorporates pure silver to safely eliminate odor-causing bacteria while keeping you cooler in the summer and warmer in the winter. In other words, you can wear one X-Static outfit for a week and not have to wash it because it doesn't hold any of your smell. It also helps control your body's core temperature when you're working out so you don't get overheated.

- **Cocona.** This fabric is made through a process that involves heating coconut shells into activated carbon, which is then fused into polyester fibers. The process results in a material that keeps you dry and cool, resists odor, and protects you from UV rays.

- **Icefil.** The fibers of this fabric cool your skin by absorbing the heat you generate while exercising and removing sweaty moisture. It also protects you from UV rays.

- **Lightning Dry.** Made from special polyester fibers, this fabric absorbs moisture and helps keep your skin dry. It is also very comfortable.

- **Bamboo.** Bamboo fibers are some of the greatest breakthroughs in fitness apparel. Its features include breathability and antimicrobial protection. For the environmentally conscious, bamboo is a highly renewal resource that grows quickly and is harvested for many types of green products.

- **Nylon.** This old favorite still works well. It is excellent for its anti-abrasive properties and breathability.

Garments with Give

Buy garments that have a bit of stretch (spandex content, elastic waist) to them. Also look for bottoms that have a drawstring waist, adjustable features, or a roll-down waist so you can easily adjust it to your weight loss. Hosiery and tights infused with spandex tone and firms legs and thighs in a nanosecond. Choose pantyhose with a built-in support brief to slim down that tummy and tush.

Makeup to the Rescue!

No matter where you are in your weight-loss journey—pounds away from your goal or close to it—there is yet another way to look five pounds thinner in minutes without slashing calories or sweating: makeup. Use these tricks of the trade to dramatically slim down your face and body:

- Help fade puffiness and dark circles. Try to get enough sleep each night (between eight and nine hours), which can help minimize shadows and puffiness. Also, look for gentle eye creams that contain vitamin K and the natural skin-lighteners kojic acid and licorice extract. Some experts believe dark circles are caused by veins and capillaries showing through the thin undereye skin. That's why vitamin K, which helps constrict capillaries, seems to help.

- Use contouring to make your face appear thinner. Apply your blush below your cheekbone. You can also apply a bronzing powder on either side of your throat to extend the lines of your neck. Bring out the angles in your face by highlighting them. Use an iridescent cream or powder along the tops of your cheekbones and blend well. You can take this one step further by blending the same iridescent shimmer along your collarbone. Do not put your blush on the apples of your cheeks unless you want to look fatter. Blush should be put where the jaw and skull meet; the natural line of your cheek is where you should put blush. To identify the right spot, pinch your cheeks in, revealing the contour of the cheekbone

- Get a thinner-looking face by shaping your eyebrows correctly. Beautifully sculpted brows frame the eyes, add definition to the face, and draw attention to the middle. Make sure yours are tweezed, waxed, lasered, or otherwise groomed.

- Use a self-tanner or bronzer. A good tan can make you look thinner. If you use a tanning lotion, use more under the cheeks, as the colored areas will look deeper. That will make your face look thinner than it really is. Dark color makes areas recede, so use bronzer—either liquid or powder—below your cheekbones, along the jaw line, and under the chin. Be extra sure that everything is very well blended so you don't look like you're wearing a dark mask.

- Make your eyes look as big as possible. The larger they look in proportion to the rest of your face, the more petite your face will seem overall. Lightly dust a pale, shimmery shadow from your lash line to your brow bone. Brush a neutral taupe or gray into the crease. Line your eyes across the entire upper lash line, and instead of eyeliner on the bottom lashes, dab a bit of taupe or brown shadow into the lash line for a softer look. Curl your lashes and use two coats of volumizing mascara, making sure you let it dry between coats. To make your eyes "pop" even more, apply false lashes to the outer corners.

- Plump up your lips with a dab of gloss directly in the middle of the lower lip. Avoid lip liner, as it can make your pout look smaller. Dab a teeny bit of bronzer or light brown eye shadow just under the center of your bottom lip, right where it folds down.

For Men Only: Look Trim and Fit in Your Clothes

My men clients want to look trimmer in their clothes, just as we women do. Here are some tips for men:

- Wear your pants correctly. Make sure they are worn at your natural waistline. They should be well fitting and loose enough to drape. Wear a belt with your pants, but don't cinch it in.

- Wear the same color shirt and pants in a medium to dark tone, perhaps with a different-colored sports coat.

- Avoid thick, bulky fabrics, which make you look bigger instead of slimmer.

- Wear lightweight fabrics and darker colors. They'll give the illusion of a smaller stomach.

- Wear long sleeves. Short-sleeved tops and T-shirts can draw attention to your stomach.

- Avoid tight-fitting clothes. They call attention to your body and make you look bigger.

- Go for vertical stripes because they make you appear slimmer.

- Stay away from loud, tropical shirts until you slim down. They call attention to a large frame.

- For business suits, gravitate toward dark-toned ones made of non-creasing fabrics for a slimming effect. Pair the same color of suit and shirt with a contrasting vest long enough to cover your belt.

- Keep your jacket buttoned to look slimmer instantly.

- Don't tuck in your shirt if you have a big stomach. Doing so will make your stomach look bigger. Keeping your shirt out camouflages your stomach, making it appear slimmer.

- Avoid baggy clothes because they make you look more bulky.

Building a wardrobe is like collecting your favorite things. Your choices should be careful and personal and should reflect your taste not just for a season but for years to come. Style is knowing yourself and what looks best on you.

Naked Fitness on the Inside

It's wonderful to have a body that is beautiful on the outside, naked, and in clothes. But what about the inside—your overall health? In addition to following a healthy lifestyle, one of the best moves you can make is to see your doctor on a regular basis for annual tests and screenings designed for your age group and sex.

Many of us take better care of our cars than our own bodies. At the first squeak or rattle, we head to the mechanic for a full check. But when our bodies show early signs of trouble, we put off visits to the doctor, not realizing that like our cars, medical checkups are vital to remain in good health.

Whether you're 15 or 50 or older, yearly checkups are part of that ounce of prevention. A routine physical ensures that your body is in good health and lets you head off any potentially serious problems.

A physical is a head-to-toe search for signs of trouble. It's typically divided into three parts: history, the exam itself, and laboratory tests. During the history, your doctor will ask you questions about allergies, medications, past illnesses, hospitalizations, and lifestyle habits that might affect your health, such as drinking, smoking, and exercise habits.

During the exam portion of the checkup, your physician moves down your body, checking that all systems are functioning properly and looking for abnormalities.

He or she tests your blood pressure, listens to your heart and lungs for irregularities, checks your eyes for clues about diabetes and high blood pressure, and checks your throat for infection or obstruction. Your doctor will examine your arms and hands for signs of neurological damage, feel your breasts for lumps, and prod your abdomen for masses or signs of disease.

Lab tests make up the last part of the physical. Routine tests such as pap smears, mammograms, and prostate, vaginal, and rectal exams are scheduled based on age, sex, and general health. Your doctor might order other tests such as X-rays, MRIs, and CAT scans based on your medical history and any physical exam findings.

Here is a brief summary of tests that are recommended as part of a complete physical. It was provided primarily by the Cleveland Clinic.

Routine Lab Tests

FASTING BLOOD SUGAR. At least one-fourth of U.S. adults are known to have prediabetes, a condition defined as having impaired fasting glucose, impaired glucose tolerance, or both. People with prediabetes are at increased risk for developing type 2 diabetes, heart disease, and stroke. The test works like this: After you have gone for at least 8 to 10 hours without food, a sample of your blood is drawn at your doctor's office and sent to a lab for analysis. After fasting, normal plasma glucose levels are less than 100 milligrams per deciliter (mg/dL). If your fasting plasma glucose levels exceed 126 mg/dL, your doctor may suspect diabetes.

FASTING LIPID PROFILE. This includes total cholesterol, HDL (good cholesterol), LDL (bad cholesterol), and triglyceride levels. (See pages 281–282 for more information.)

COMPLETE BLOOD COUNT (CBC). This blood test screens for anemia, which is caused by lower-than-normal numbers of oxygen-carrying red blood cells. Unchecked, it can lead to heart failure. It also measures levels of liver enzymes.

HIGH-SENSITIVE C-REACTIVE PROTEIN. This simple test measures the amount of inflammation in your body by examining levels of C-reactive protein (CRP) in your bloodstream. The body naturally produces an inflammatory response to fight off infections and heal wounds, but chronically high levels can cause your blood vessels to harden or fat to build up in your arteries.

Excess CRP has also been linked to the development of other problems including diabetes, high blood pressure, and Alzheimer's disease. The test is like an early warning system for your entire body. If your level is high (a score of 3 milligrams per liter or more), your physician may recommend that you exercise 30 minutes a day and increase your intake of vegetables, whole grains, and lean protein or take medications such as cholesterol-lowering statins or aspirin to fight inflammation.

VITAMIN D LEVEL. Low levels are associated with osteopenia, osteoporosis, breast cancer, colon cancer, and heart disease.

HPV ASSAY. A woman with a normal Pap smear and HPV assay can increase her intervals for screening for cervical cancer to every three years.

Tests and Screenings Recommended by Age
TWENTIES
EYE EXAM. An eye exam is the best way to protect your vision and to prevent future eye problems. It's best to have an eye check at least once a year in your 20s and twice a year in your 30s.

SKIN CHECK. It's important to have your skin checked regularly for odd-shaped or changing moles. Detecting and treating melanoma early is the key to beating the disease.

ANNUAL PELVIC EXAMS AND STD SCREENINGS. Women who have been sexually active and have a cervix should have cervical cancer screenings. Routine Pap tests should begin by age 18 or 21 for all women. Screening may be discontinued after age 65 if the woman has had three normal Pap tests in a row and no abnormal Pap smears within the last 10 years.

Several of the most common STDs, including chlamydia and human papillomavirus (HPV), often do not produce obvious symptoms but if

untreated can increase a woman's risk of cervical cancer and even infer-
tility. However, you may be able to skip a year or two if three consecutive,
annual Pap tests come back normal or if you have both the Pap and HPV
tests and both are regularly normal.

All sexually active women 25 and younger and other asymptomatic
women at increased risk for infection should have A chlamydia infection test.

All sexually active women should have a gonorrhea infection test if
they are at increased risk for infection (that is, if they are 25 or younger
or have other individual or population risk factors).

All adolescents and adults at increased risk for HIV infection should
have an HIV infection test. This includes men and women who have un-
protected sex with multiple partners, past or present injection drug users,
individuals whose past or present sex partners were HIV-infected, and
persons being treated for sexually transmitted diseases.

THIRTIES

CHOLESTEROL LEVEL. Cholesterol screening is recommended for men 35
and older, and then at least once every five years—more frequently if you
are overweight or have a family history of heart disease to detect early
warning signs. (See information on pages 281–282 on how to read these
tests.)

THYROID TEST. Your thyroid gland produces hormones that regulate the
way your body uses energy. You should get a thyroid check by age 35 to
help determine if the gland is functioning properly.

BLOOD PRESSURE. The only way to detect high blood pressure is by getting
it checked. High blood pressure can lead to heart attack, stroke, or kidney
failure, so it's important to get it tested at least once a year. Generally, a
reading of less than 120 over 80 indicates healthy blood pressure, while
a reading of 140 over 90 at the doctor's office is considered high (if taken
at home, 135 over 85 is considered high).

FORTIES

CHOLESTEROL. Cholesterol increases with age. After age 45, women should have a blood test for total cholesterol, HDL (good cholesterol), and LDL (bad cholesterol). Women and men younger than the stated age may be screened if they have other risk factors for heart disease. Here is a look at how to interpret your results:

Total Blood (or Serum) Cholesterol Level
Less than 200 mg/dL: Normal
200 to 239 mg/dL: Borderline high
240 mg/dL and over: High

HDL (Good) Cholesterol
With HDL (good) cholesterol, higher levels are better. Low HDL cholesterol (less than 40 mg/dL for men, less than 50 mg/dL for women) puts you at higher risk for heart disease. In the average man, HDL cholesterol levels range from 40 to 50 mg/dL. In the average woman, they range from 50 to 60 mg/dL. An HDL cholesterol level of 60 mg/dL or higher provides some protection against heart disease.

LDL (Bad) Cholesterol
The lower your LDL cholesterol, the lower your risk of heart attack and stroke. In fact, it's a better gauge of risk than total blood cholesterol. In general, LDL levels fall into the following categories.

LDL Cholesterol Levels
Less than 100 mg/dL   Optimal
100 to 129 mg/dL   Near optimal/above optimal
130 to 159 mg/dL   Borderline high
160 to 189 mg/dL   High
190 mg/dL and above   Very high

Triglyceride Level
Your triglyceride level will fall into one of these categories:
Less than 150 mg/dL: Normal
150–199 mg/dL: Borderline high
200–499 mg/dL: High
500 mg/dL: Very High

EYE TESTS. Catch signs of glaucoma, age-related macular degeneration, and cataracts. A yearly glaucoma test includes two tests that are often given at annual eye exams: tonometry and ophthalmoscopy. During a tonometry, your doctor measures the inner pressure of the eye with a puff of air or a probe. Ophthalmoscopy is used to examine the inside of the eye. The doctor will use a lighted instrument to examine the optic nerve.

MAMMOGRAM. Breast cancer screening should include a mammogram every one to two years for women 40 and older.

FIFTIES

PROSTATE CANCER SCREENING. Most physicians recommend prostate cancer screening for men age 50 to 70 and for men over 45 who have an increased risk. This consists of a blood test for prostate-specific antigen (PSA) or a digital rectal exam. Generally, if the PSA is more than 10 ng/mL, the patient has even odds of having cancer. The gray area lies between 4 and 10 ng/mL. Less than 4 is desirable.

COLONOSCOPY. The risk of colon cancer—the fourth most common cancer in women and men—increases with age. It's often curable if detected early. Colorectal cancer screening, preferably with a colonoscopy, should be done in men and women 50 years or older. If you had a parent or sibling who had colon cancer before age 60, screening might start sooner. Colonoscopy is the best test for detecting cancer and larger polyps but has slightly higher risks than other tests.

BONE-DENSITY (DEXA) SCAN. Estrogen levels plummet as you age, increasing your risk for osteopenia, or low bone mass, which can lead to osteoporosis if not treated. Often called a DEXA scan, this low-radiation X-ray assesses your risk of developing osteoporosis and osteopenia. Caused by low levels of calcium and other minerals in your bones, these conditions weaken bones over time, making them vulnerable to fractures.

You need this test if you smoke, have a family history of fractures, or have suffered from an eating disorder. Although women typically don't think about osteoporosis until after menopause, if you have low bone density, you can take preventive measures now,

Routine screening should begin at age 60 for women at increased risk for fractures. Screening should be repeated every two to three years to detect changes in bone density.

SIXTIES

AORTIC ANEURYSM. A one-time screening for abdominal aortic aneurysm (bulging wall of the aorta in the abdomen) should be performed by ultrasound in men age 65 to 75 who have ever smoked.

DIABETES. Diabetes affects more than 23 million Americans, increases their risk of heart disease and stroke, and can lead to kidney disease and blindness. Anyone with risk behaviors should request this test. A relatively new, little known, benefit from Medicare offers free screenings to most people over 65. Less than 10 percent of those who qualify for it take advantage of it.

HEARING. At least 30 percent of people over 60 have some hearing loss, most of which is treatable. During the exam, you'll be asked to react to different noises by repeating words and responding to various pitches. If you have hearing loss, you'll be referred to an ear, nose, and throat specialist for an examination to pinpoint the exact cause: Benign tumors, ear infections, or a perforated ear drum can all be culprits. If your loss is permanent, you can be fitted for hearing aids. Get a hearing test at least once every three years.

OTHER TESTS

Depression screening is recommended for all adults and involves asking a few simple questions.

Your physician may recommend the following tests if you have symptoms or a family history:

- Bladder cancer screening with a urine analysis
- Breast cancer susceptibility gene testing for women without a family history of increased risk
- Lung cancer screening with a chest X-ray if you are smoker
- Ovarian cancer screening with blood tests or ultrasound
- Pancreas cancer screening with blood tests or ultrasound
- Testicular cancer screening by clinical examination
- Coronary heart disease screening with EKG, exercise stress test, or CT scan for coronary calcium in adults with low or increased risk of heart disease
- Hepatitis B and C screening

Please keep in mind that these are general guidelines, and each patient requires a specific analysis of his or her risk factors that will help the physician determine the appropriate screening tests.

Naked Fitness: Steps to My Healthy Body

In the space below, describe what you want your body to look like and feel like:

_____

_____

_____

_____

_____

_____

_____

_____

_____

_____

_____

Write down the steps necessary to make this happen. These might include losing 15 pounds, exercising more, learning to rock climb, eating more vegetables, making Naked Fitness your lifestyle, or all of the above.

_____

_____

_____

_____

_____

_____

_____

_____

_____

_____

_____

_____

_____

_____

Naked Fitness: Standing in the Mirror Naked

Strip Away the Problems to Look Better Naked

List at least 5 things that are holding you back or have contributed to missing the mark.

List why this time it will be different. Draw from your past when you have overcome this.

1. _____

_____

2. _____

_____

3. _____

_____

4. _____

_____

5. _____

_____

1. _____

_____

2. _____

_____

3. _____

_____

4. _____

_____

5. _____

_____

Why I will look better naked. (List the people who will support you, time you can put into your schedule, and other items that will build your success.)

People   **Time**   **Other**

_____

_____

_____

_____

_____

_____

_____

_____

_____

_____

_____

_____

_____

_____

_____

_____

My success story—Opening my own fitness studio

Describe your success story: I decided to open my own business. I had to chart out a business plan- like a worksheet. I had to decide how much time I would be willing to invest into the plan. I had to decide how much money I was going put into the studio and what my return would be. I had to train staff and be creative with how to market, set up, schedule, and attain new clients. I had to use my network of friends to help organize the studio and have them volunteer their time in exchange for free fitness classes and studio usage to have a front desk presence. I had to order equipment, train friends that seemed like they had good personal skills and an understanding of the body to be personal trainers. I had to work at this job everyday to make it happen and didn't see any results until three months of preparation before we opened the studio. I had to multi-task activities and still find time to balance out my personal, family and financial life during the process. MBC Fitness is located in downtown Westmont since 2002 at 28 N Cass Avenue, www.mbcftitness.com

Now look at your success. What are some words you would use that describe what you accomplished (i.e., perseverance, discipline, etc.)? List as many of these words as possible. Of course I see many words: scheduling, finding time to balance, discipline, seeking information and researching, trying new things, learning new computer skills, learning about marketing, reading books on marketing, business plans and fitness, outgoing, support network, daily work on this job, waking up earlier to train people than head to work to the studio to change it. Drawing out a big plan.

Now what is your goal? Losing weight, lowering your cholesterol, starting an exercise program? What do you need to do to be your best, healthiest, naked self? My goal for a healthier lifestyle: Being a role model that exercises every day and helps create programs to get others to find that sense of balance and health a little easier to accomplish. I have many goals for myself . . . eating better, sleeping better, exercising daily, and working on my own alignment, and posture. I commit to making this happen!

Your success story

Describe your success story:

_____

_____

_____

_____

_____

_____

Now look at your success. What are some words you would use that describe what you accomplished (i.e., perseverance, discipline, etc.)? List as many of these words as possible.

_____

_____

_____

_____

Now what is your goal? Losing weight, lowering your cholesterol, starting an exercise program? What do you need to do to be your best, healthiest, naked self?

_____

_____

_____

_____

Naked Fitness: Daily Walking Log

Monday	Tuesday	Wednesday	Thursday
Date:	Date:	Date:	Date:
Miles:	Miles:	Miles:	Miles:
Steps:	Steps:	Steps:	Steps:
Time:	Time:	Time:	Time:

Friday	Saturday	Sunday	Total
Date:	Date:	Date:	
Miles:	Miles:	Miles:	
Steps:	Steps:	Steps:	
Time:	Time:	Time:	

Monday	Tuesday	Wednesday	Thursday
Date:	Date:	Date:	Date:
Miles:	Miles:	Miles:	Miles:
Steps:	Steps:	Steps:	Steps:
Time:	Time:	Time:	Time:

Friday	Saturday	Sunday	Total
Date:	Date:	Date:	
Miles:	Miles:	Miles:	
Steps:	Steps:	Steps:	
Time:	Time:	Time:	

Monday	**Tuesday**	**Wednesday**	**Thursday**
Date:	Date:	Date:	Date:
Miles:	Miles:	Miles:	Miles:
Steps:	Steps:	Steps:	Steps:
Time:	Time:	Time:	Time:

Friday	**Saturday**	**Sunday**	**Total**
Date:	Date:	Date:	
Miles:	Miles:	Miles:	
Steps:	Steps:	Steps:	
Time:	Time:	Time:	

Monday	**Tuesday**	**Wednesday**	**Thursday**
Date:	Date:	Date:	Date:
Miles:	Miles:	Miles:	Miles:
Steps:	Steps:	Steps:	Steps:
Time:	Time:	Time:	Time:

Friday	**Saturday**	**Sunday**	**Total**
Date:	Date:	Date:	
Miles:	Miles:	Miles:	
Steps:	Steps:	Steps:	
Time:	Time:	Time:	

Naked Fitness Recipes

NAKED FITNESS POLENTA CHILI

5 chicken sausages (the entire package)
Polenta, 18-oz. package
Salsa, one 12-oz. jar
Garbanzo beans (chickpeas), one 15-oz. can, rinsed and drained

Start the grill. Grill the chicken sausage until done and then chop it into small pieces. Next, chop the packaged polenta in small pieces and put it in a pot with 1½ cups boiling water until it becomes creamy. Add the salsa, rinsed garbanzo beans, and chicken sausage. Heat thoroughly. Divide into five 2-cup servings.

NAKED FITNESS TORTILLA SOUP

1 cup carrots, diced
1 cup onions, diced
8 cups chicken stock
8 tortillas, chopped into ¼-inch strips
Salsa, 1 12-oz. jar
Black beans, 1 15-oz. can, rinsed and drained
Fajita seasoning, 1 packet
Cilantro, ½ cup fresh chopped

Salt to taste
Pepper to taste
2 cups chopped grilled chicken

Put a soup pot on the stove and lightly oil with either cooking spray or small drops of olive oil and wipe with paper towel to coat. Add the carrots and onions and cook for 3 to 4 minutes. Next add the chicken stock and tortillas pieces. Bring to a boil and let cook for 20 minutes or until tortillas dissolve in the soup. Add the salsa, rinsed beans, fajita seasoning packet, and cilantro. Add salt and pepper to taste. Add 2 cups chopped grilled chicken breast. Separate into 5 servings.

NAKED FITNESS EGGS ASPARAGUS

12 eggs
1 bunch asparagus, chopped
¼ cup skim milk
2 roma tomatoes (each sliced into 6 pieces)
4 tsp. salt-free seasoning
1 cup parmesan cheese
4 green onions, chopped

Lightly beat together eggs, milk, salt-free seasoning, and ¾ cup parmesan cheese. Pour into a nonstick sprayed or lightly oiled 12×6×2-inch glass or ceramic baking dish coated with nonstick cooking spray. Sprinkle in onions and then asparagus. Layer on the sliced tomatoes, and then sprinkle the remaining parmesan on the top. Bake, uncovered, at 350°F for 40 to 45 minutes until puffy in the center and lightly browned or until a knife inserted near the center comes out clean. Let stand 5 minutes before serving. Makes 4 servings (3 for you and 1 for a friend or for beginning your next week).

BUTTERNUT CRAB BISQUE

3 cups butternut squash
4 cups chicken stock
Curry powder, salt, and pepper to taste
8 oz. jumbo lump crab meat (canned)

Cut the butternut squash in half lengthwise. Place half of it in the microwave for about 6 to 8 minutes. Scoop out the seeds and discard. Scoop out the flesh and puree it. Add the pureed squash to the chicken stock and bring to a boil. Add curry powder. Pour into bowls. Add 4 oz. lump crab meat to each bowl and serve. Makes 2 servings.

CHICKEN PATTIES

4 cups cooked shredded chicken
1 cup shredded cheddar cheese
2 eggs
½ cup chopped onion
2 cloves minced garlic
4 tbsp. organic flaxseed meal
Seasoning to taste

Shred cooked chicken breast. To the chicken, add the cheddar cheese, onion, minced garlic, and flax. Form into six patties. Spray a cookie sheet with vegetable cooking spray and place patties on cookie sheet. Lightly spray patties (about ½ second on each one) Bake at 375°F for 15 minutes. Makes 6 servings.

TURKEY BACON CHEESE FRITTATA

8 large eggs
½ cup nonfat milk
4 tablespoons fresh cilantro, chopped
2 tbsp. olive oil
4 slices turkey bacon, cooked

1 medium white onion, chopped
2 medium tomatoes, one diced, one sliced
4 oz. low-fat grated white cheddar cheese
Garlic powder and black pepper to taste

Chop turkey bacon into small pieces. To the bacon, add chopped onion and sauté until onions are brown. Turn off heat and stir in chopped tomato. Let the mixture sit.

Beat eggs and skim milk in a small bowl. Add chopped cilantro (and garlic powder and pepper if desired). Heat olive oil in a skillet over medium heat for about 2 minutes. Pour in the egg mixture. Once the egg mixture is almost firm, add the sautéed mixture to the center of the omelet. Next, add the cheese and fold the edges over the center. Garnish with additional cilantro and sliced tomato. Makes 4 servings.

HUMMUS, TURKEY, AND AVOCADO WRAPS

1 25-oz. jar hummus
½ tsp. kosher salt
¼ tsp. black pepper
6 low-carbohydrate tortillas, 10-inch
1 small red onion, thinly sliced
1 cucumber, preferably hothouse (seedless), thinly sliced (peeled, if desired)
1 4- to 5-oz. container sprouts (alfalfa, radish, broccoli, or a combination)
2 avocados, pitted and thinly sliced
24 oz. sliced turkey lunchmeat

Place tortillas on a work surface. Divide hummus evenly on the tortillas. Top with the onion, cucumber, sprouts, avocado, and 4 oz. of turkey. You can make these each morning or just add the sprouts to a premade one, and they will keep nicely. Makes 6 servings.

ARTICHOKE AND BEEF LETTUCE WRAPS

1 13-oz. can of artichokes, rinsed and sliced
½ lb. roast beef thinly sliced
1 13-oz. can of garbanzo beans, rinsed and drained
¼ cup packed fresh basil
2 tsp. capers, chopped
¼ cup lemon juice
1 tsp. olive oil
Dash of salt and pepper
16 romaine lettuce leaves

Place artichokes, beef, garbanzos, parmesan, basil, capers, lemon juice, and oil in a bowl and mix. Sprinkle with salt and pepper. Put ¼ cup of this filling in each romaine leaf. You can refrigerate the mixture and assemble them at lunchtime. Makes 4 servings of 4 wraps each.

WRAPPED-UP PIZZA SALAD

3 tomatoes, chopped
¼ cup red onion, diced
¼ cup chicken broth (reduced sodium)
2 tbsp. red wine vinegar
Dash of salt and pepper
1 cup mini-cubed low fat skim mozzarella cheese
1 cup roasted red peppers, thinly sliced
¼ cup turkey pepperoni, thinly sliced
¼ cup chopped packed basil
8 low-carbohydrate tortillas, 10-inch

Mix all ingredients, except tortillas, and refrigerate 1 hour. Evenly divide into the tortillas. Makes 4 servings or 2 wraps each.

NAKED FITNESS SMOOTHIE

½ cup protein powder, chocolate flavor
3 almonds
½ banana
2 cups ice

Blend all ingredients together and enjoy as a snack.

Naked Fitness: Maintenance Strategies

It's important to record strategies you'll employ to stay lean and fit. Please make some notes here.

_____

_____

_____

_____

I do not want to regain my weight because:

_____

_____

_____

_____

The following Naked Fitness tools worked best for me:

_____

_____

_____

_____

Obstacles I need to keep stripping away are:

_____

_____

_____

_____

I will strip these away by:

_____

_____

_____

_____

If my weight starts climbing up again, I will: (figure out if its due to a change in eating or exercise, bigger portions, less walking, slipping into bad habits, etc.)

_____

_____

_____

_____

I will take the following actions if I regain weight:

_____

_____

_____

_____

Naked Fitness:
Charting My Day: The Time Wasters

The purpose of this chart is to help you map out an entire day. In each box write as many things as you can remember about your daily activities. Circle the most important and redline the least important. Your redlined items represent minutes you can potentially free up.

Early Morning

Mid-Morning

Lunchtime

Mid-Afternoon

Dinnertime

Evening

Naked Fitness: Food Journal

Day/Date:

Meal	Food and Beverages	Place	Calories	How I felt

Day/Date:

Meal	Food and Beverages	Place	Calories	How I felt

Useful Websites

Naked Fitness (www.nakedfitness.com)
   Support material for this book
Andrea Metcalf (www.andreametcalf.com)
   Information on my various programs
Calorie King (www.calorieking.com)
   An interactive website where you can look up the calorie count of
   virtually any food
Everyday Health (www.everydayhealth.com)
   Information on health, diseases, and medication. Also provides meal
   planners, a symptom checker, and a physician locator
FitnessConnect (www.fitnessconnect.com)
   A website listing certified trainers in your area from the most presti-
   gious certifying agencies
U.S. Department of Health and Human Services (HHS)
(www.health.gov)
   A portal to the websites of a number of multiagency health initiatives
   and activities of the HHS)
Health Steps RX (www.healthstepsrx.com)
   Information and interactive help on weight control and diabetes
   management
Kid's Health (www.kidshealth.org)
   Information for kids and teens on all aspects of health
About.Com: Longevity (www.longevity.about.com)
   Information on anti-aging

Real Age (www.realage.com)

    An interactive website where you can calculate your "real age" based on your health and lifestyle habits

Paws-ilates™ (www.pawsilates.com)

    A Pilates exercise program for you and your dog

Sparks People (www.sparkspeople.com)

    Personalized diet and fitness plans

Surgeon General (www.surgeongeneral.gov)

    A government website with links to websites and information related to the Surgeon General's office.

Walk Jog Run (www.walkjogrun.net)

    A free and easy way to create running routes or find one from the organization's member running routes

WebMD (www.webmd.com)

    Informative website on all aspects of health, wellness, and disease management

Naked Fitness Bibliography

Barlow, J. 2001. Consuming more protein, fewer carbohydrates may be healthier. Press release, News Bureau, University of Illinois at Urbana-Champaign.

Bocalini, D.S. et al. 2008. Water-versus land-based exercise effects on physical fitness in older women. *Geriatrics & Gerontology International* 8:265–271.

Brooks, B.M. et al. 2006. Association of calcium intake, dairy product consumption with overweight status in young adults (1995-1996): the Bogalusa Heart Study. *Journal of the American College of Nutrition* 25:523–532.

Catenacci, V.A. et al. 2008. Physical activity patterns in the National Weight Control Registry. *Obesity* 16:153–161.

deBusk, R.F. et al. 1990. Training effects of long versus short bouts of exercise in healthy subjects. *American Journal of Cardiology* 65: 1010–1013.

de Oliveira, M.C. et al. 2008. A low-energy-dense diet adding fruit reduces weight and energy intake in women. *Appetite* 51:291–295.

Editor. 2008. Sitting all day can be hazardous to your health. *Current Cardiovascular Risk Results*, July.

En-Ting, C. 2009. The impact of daytime naps on the relation between sleep duration and cardiovascular events. *Archives of Internal Medicine* 169:717.

Fogelholm, M. et al. 2000. Effects of walking training on weight maintenance after a very-low-energy diet in premenopausal obese women: a randomized controlled trial. *Archives of Internal Medicine* 24:2177–2184.

Geneviève, C. et al. 2009. Calcium plus vitamin D supplementation and fat mass loss in female very low-calcium consumers: potential link with a calcium-specific appetite control. *British Journal of Nutrition* 101:659–663.

Gilhooly, C.H. et al. 2007. Food cravings and energy regulation: the characteristics of craved foods and their relationship with eating behaviors and weight change during 6 months of dietary energy restriction. *International Journal of Obesity* 31:1849–1858.

Howarth, N.C. et al. 2001. Dietary fiber and weight regulation. *Nutrition Review* 59:129–139.

Jennings, A.E. et al. 2009. The effect of exercise training on resting metabolic rate in Type 2 Diabetes Mellitus. *Medicine & Science in Sports & Exercise* 41(8):1558–1565.

Johnson, R.W. 2009. Neighborhood food environment and walkability predict obesity in New York City. Mailman School of Public Health, Columbia University, New York.

King, A.C. et al. 1997. Moderate-intensity exercise and self-rated quality of sleep in older adults. A randomized controlled trial. *Journal of the American Medical Association* 277:32–37.

Kohrt, W.M. et al. 1992. Exercise training improves fat distribution patterns in 60 to 70-year-old men and women. *Journal of Gerontology* 47:M99–105.

Kripke, D.F. et. al 2002. Mortality associated with sleep duration and insomnia. *Archives of General Psychiatry* 59(2):137–138.

LeBlanc, J. et al. 1993. Components of postprandial thermogenesis in relation to meal frequency in humans. *Canadian Journal of Physiology Pharmacology* 71:879–883.

Lee, Y.H. et al. 2010. Effect of glucosamine or chondroitin sulfate on the osteoarthritis progression: a meta-analysis. *Rheumatology International* 30:357–363.

Manson, J.E. et al. 1999. A prospective study of walking as compared with vigorous exercise in the prevention of coronary heart disease in women. *New England Journal of Medicine* 341:650.

McManus, K. et al. 2001. A randomized controlled trial of a moderate-fat, low-energy diet compared with a low fat, low-energy diet for weight loss in overweight adults. International *Journal of Obesity and Metabolism Related Disorders* 25:1503–1511.

Norman, T.M, et al. 2010. Efficacy of a progressive walking program and glucosamine sulphate supplementation on osteoarthritic symptoms of the hip and knee: a feasibility trial. *Arthritis Research and Therapy* 12:R25.

Petersen, S.G. et al. 2010. Glucosamine but not ibuprofen alters cartilage turnover in osteoarthritis patients in response to physical training. *Osteoarthritis and Cartilage* 18:34–40.

Roberts, S.B. et al. 2002. The influence of dietary composition on energy intake and body weight. *Journal of the American College of Nutrition* 21:140S–145S.

Rodgers, C.D. et. al. 1995. Energy expenditure during submaximal walking with Exerstriders. *Medicine & Science in Sports & Exercise* 27(4).

Rolls, B.J. et al. 1997. Is the low-fat message giving people a license to eat more? *Journal of the American College of Nutrition* 16:535–543.

Rolls, B.J. et al. 2002. Portion size of food affects energy intake in normal-weight and overweight men and women. *American Journal of Clinical Nutrition* 76:1207–1213.

Schulze, M.B. et al. 2004. Sugar-sweetened beverages, weight gain, and incidence of type 2 diabetes in young and middle-aged women. *Journal of the American Medical Association* 292:927–934.

Skov, A.R. et al. 1999. Randomized trial on protein vs carbohydrate in ad libitum fat reduced diet for the treatment of obesity. *International Journal of Obesity and Metabolism Related Disorders* 23:528–536.

Sun, Q. et al. 2010. Physical activity at midlife in relation to successful survival in women at age 70 years or older. *Archives of Internal Medicine* 170:194–201.

Taheri, S. et al. 2004. Short sleep duration is associated with reduced leptin, elevated ghrelin, and increased body mass index. *PLoS Medicine* 1:e62.

Vander Wal, J.S. et al. 2005. Short-term effect of eggs on satiety in overweight and obese subjects. *Journal of the American College of Nutrition* 24:510–515.

VanWormer, J.J. et al. 2008. Self-weighing promotes weight loss for obese adults. *American Journal of Preventive Medicine* 36:70–73.

Wang, S.X. et al. 2002. Effects of sleep deprivation on gamma-amino-butyric acid and glutamate contents in rat brain. *Archives of General Psychiatry* 59(2):131–136.

Weigle, D.S. et al. 2005. A high-protein diet induces sustained reductions in appetite, ad libitum caloric intake, and body weight despite compensatory changes in diurnal plasma leptin and ghrelin concentrations. *American Journal of Clinical Nutrition* 82:41–48.

Wing, R.R. et al. 2001. Successful weight loss maintenance. *Annual Review of Nutrition* 21:323–341.

Wyatt, H.R. et al. 2002. Long-term weight loss and breakfast in subjects in the National Weight Control Registry. *Obesity Research* 10: 78–82.

Yoshioka, M. et al. 1998. Effects of red pepper added to high-fat and high-carbohydrate meals on energy metabolism and substrate utilization in Japanese women. *British Journal of Nutrition* 80: 503–510.

Zemel, M.B. et al. 2005. Dairy augmentation of total and central fat loss in obese subjects. *International Journal of Obesity* 29:391–397.

Zemel, M.B. et al. 2005. Effects of calcium and dairy on body composition and weight loss in African-American adults. *Obesity Research* 13(7):1218–1225.

INDEX